Pioneering Hematology

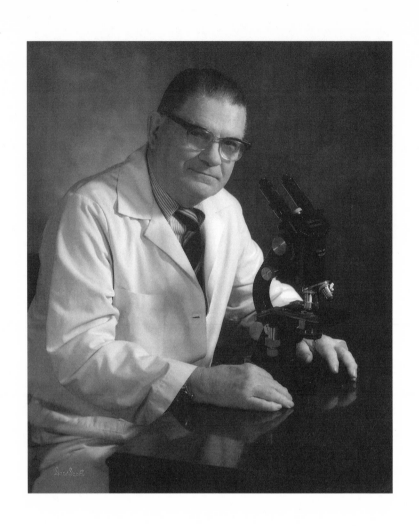

Pioneering Hematology

The research and treatment of
malignant blood disorders—
Reflections on a life's work

William C. Moloney, M.D.
and Sharon Johnson

The Francis A. Countway Library of Medicine, Boston
1997

ISBN: 0-88135-195-4

Sole distributor: Science History Publications/USA, a division of Watson
Publishing International, Canton, Massachusetts 02021-0493, U.S.A.

Dedicated to
my mother
Elizabeth Curry Moloney

CONTENTS

ILLUSTRATIONS   ix

PREFACE by H. Franklin Bunn   XI

ACKNOWLEDGMENTS   XIV

CHAPTER ONE
    Getting Started   1

CHAPTER TWO
    Cigar Box Hematology   23

CHAPTER THREE
    A "Pathologist" Goes to War   33

CHAPTER FOUR
    Hematology on the Home Front   61

CHAPTER FIVE
My Troubles With Radiation 90

CHAPTER SIX
Rats, Hawks and Doves 115

CHAPTER SEVEN
Legal Fallout 136

CHAPTER EIGHT
Under the House Calls 143

CHAPTER NINE
Cowbarns and Cathouses 152

CHAPTER TEN
Chemotherapy in the Corridors 164

CHAPTER ELEVEN
From Heyday to Mayday 177

INDEX 187

ILLUSTRATIONS

Frontispiece: William C. Moloney, photographed in 1981

Following page 114

1. William C. Moloney with mother, 1938
2. WCM during senior year at Tufts Medical School, 1932
3. WCM in 1931, with children he delivered at St. Mary's Infant Asylum, while a medical student
4. WCM on ambulance duty at Kings County Hospital, Brooklyn, 1932
5. WCM with wife Josephine, 1932
6. The Kings County house officers, 1932
7. WCM with a 23-year-old patient with Friedreich's ataxia, 1932
8. WCM deplaning in England, 1944, prior to the invasion of Europe
9. The Moloney family posed for a passport picture, 1952
10. Hiroshima, pictured at the time of the Moloneys arrival, 1952
11. A typical street in Nagasaki

12. The Atomic Bomb Casualty Commission's laboratory in Nagasaki
13. Patsy and Elizabeth Moloney in Japanese costume, 1952
14. British Medical College VIPs "checking us out"
15. Japanese party in honor of John Morin
16. Tax Cornell in the parisitology laboratory of the Atomic Bomb Casualty Commission
17. Rounds at the Atomic Bomb Casualty Commission, Hiroshima
18. Rounds with the Royal Army Medical Corps
19. Teaching award presented to WCM by the Royal Army Medical Corps
20. WCM making an "under the house" call in the Marshall Islands, 1962
21. WCM becomes Director of Laboratories at Boston City Hospital, 1954
22. WCM pictured with staff of the Harvard Unit at the Boston City Hospital during presentation ceremonies
23. The staff of the Tufts Hematology Lab, 1964–1965
24. WCM with the Bunn family at a Fenway Park baseball game, 1995

PREFACE

THIS ENTERTAINING book gives us a richly detailed account of a gifted and giving physician and his odyssey from general practice in the 1930s to contemporary high-powered academic medicine. Through his travels and adventures, we get to know Dr. Moloney and what motivated him to become one of medicine's pioneers. Although the chapters take us around the world, his Boston experiences are no less interesting. We get to know a man whose energy, intellect and love of medical discovery enabled him to leave his imprint on a broad range of disciplines–hematology, laboratory medicine, pathology, blood banking and radiation biology. Equally impressive and equally well conveyed in these pages are his character, his personality and his sense of self and his God-given role in society. As much fulfillment as he had in helping to bring medical science into the forefront, he never lost sight of his priorities–his patients and their problems came first.

This book commands the reader's interest from beginning to end. Many of the anecdotes within this narrative resonate strongly with the collective impressions of those who know and revere Bill Moloney. The book gives us a glimpse into his roots—the beguiling charm of his Irish heritage, and the strength given to him by his mother and by his Christian faith. We get an inkling of Dr. Moloney's powerful and wide-ranging intellect. He reads more serious books in a month than all of his junior hematology colleagues at the Brigham collectively read in a year! No one has more zest for life and living. Bill's love of sports both as a spectator and until very recently as a participant is a significant part of his persona, as is his penchant for hearty meals and high-spirited discourse with his countless friends. I first got to know Bill during my fellowship training in the mid 1960s at Boston City Hospital. Since then he has been a wonderfully congenial sparring partner, both on the tennis court and at the dinner table. Our friendship has greatly enriched my professional and personal life.

It is impossible to think of a medical colleague more admired, more respected, more beloved. He has trained two generations of able hematologists, all of whom are in his debt. In a casual social encounter in any of the Boston suburbs, it is commonplace to meet lay persons who know Dr. Moloney as a physician to them or to a member of their family. In the autumn of his career, over a fifteen year period, he had no fewer than five ceremonial dinners in his honor. During the inevitable roasting he gave as good as he got. No one is a better story teller, as this book amply attests.

Harvard Medical School is blessed with other men and women who have achieved greatness through their research, and even more who have made their mark because of their love of teaching and/or their devotion to their patients. A few are memorable because of their style–the force of their personality, the sharpness of their wit. Bill Moloney has it all. He is both a great man and a great guy.

H. Franklin Bunn

ACKNOWLEDGMENTS

THIS BOOK WOULD not have been written were it not for the constant urging of Frank and Betsy Bunn. Whenever the opportunity presented itself, and sometimes when it did not, Betsy would ask "When are you going to write your book, Bill?"

Thus started an eighteen-month saga between Sharon Johnson and myself, an often reluctant dragon. Fortunately, Sharon is not only an outstanding writer, but she also has a mischievous and lively sense of humor, which has seen us through some occasional tense moments. Whatever style and elegance there is belongs to Sharon. But without Richard Wolfe, the task would have been impossible. Dick has been a friend in need. His expertise and knowledge have been indispensable.

My friends and associates have been kind, helpful and supportive. In addition to Frank and Betsy Bunn, David Rosenthal, Jane Desforges, Ronald McCaffery, and Hal Churchill deserve special mention.

While the stories are unique to me, the experiences

surrounding them are not. I hope this book represents the thoughts and feelings of many of my colleagues, all of whom shared a deep and fundamental dedication to patient care. I am heartened to recognize that this caring spirit and sense of commitment persists in the younger generation of physicians. I wish them godspeed as they continue to charge the medical horizon and pioneer new territory.

William C. Moloney
Chatham, Massachusetts
July, 1997

Chapter One

GETTING STARTED

1907–1934

THE DAY I left Boston City Hospital my fellows and co-workers presented me with a blue, leather-bound album. The title, "A Hematological Cookbook," was embossed in gold on the front cover. Inside were 144 hand-typed pages of "recipes" we routinely used to concoct various types of blood tests and chemotherapy combinations. "Dr. Moloney, this is your life," they joked as they handed it to me. In a way they were right. Those recipes represent a lifetime's worth of accumulation, and each one carries with it a story and a memory: the day Robin Coombs showed me how to do his newly-discovered Coombs test; the patient who responded well to a particular therapy and lived long enough to go on her honeymoon; the young fellow who stood by my side and took meticulous notes as I showed him how to do a bone marrow aspiration. It is those stories, not the recipes themselves, that really represent my life as a hematologist. Some of them are recorded here.

As a child growing up in Charlestown, I was no stranger to blood. I got in my share of fights, and could tell you the story of my childhood from the scars on my face. It was a tough town. I had to fight my way to get to school and back again. I broke my arm three times. The scar on my forehead came from a coasting accident and the scar on the back of my neck came courtesy of a Chelsea kid who chased me to my front door and hit me with a bottle. I was eleven at the time.

We were not rich and we weren't poor, and we had some intellectual background. My mother's brother was a pathologist on the Harvard faculty, which was unusual for the neighborhood. She taught me the value of reading, and every afternoon before allowing me to go outside and play, insisted I study my Latin. "People who go to Harvard read Latin," she said by way of explanation.

Yet, as things turned out, people who read Latin do not always graduate from Boston Latin School. I entered in seventh grade, in 1919, and that first year I did not pass. I simply had no interest in studying. But my mother's plans for me would not be thwarted. She grabbed me by the scruff of the neck and said, "You're going to learn Caesar." And by God I did. I was there with Tom, my middle brother. This affiliation did not enhance my reputation at Latin. Tom smoked cigars in the locker room on a regular basis, and once stayed behind during a fire drill and nailed down the tops of all the desks. The headmaster said, "Mrs. Moloney, your boys are not the Latin School type." She pulled us both out and enrolled us in the local Jamaica Plain High School. Much to my dismay, she still insisted I continue with my Latin studies.

As Catholics we had to go to Mass every Sunday. At least we were supposed to. Sunday was the day mother would unwind the tight bun she wore all week and brush her hair. Her hair was extremely long, and she'd never quite finish in time to get us to Mass. Instead, she'd take us over to Franklin Park, where we'd kneel down and say our prayers. Reflecting back, it seems I grew up in somewhat of a Dickensonian atmosphere. Just look at the institutions operating at the time. There was St. Mary's Infant Asylum, The Home for Destitute Catholic Children, The Boston Home for the Insane, The Rose Lathrop Home for the Cancerous Poor. Two or three times per year orphans would be brought into church and lined up in front for all to see. "Can anyone take these children in?" the Father would ask. Remarkably, parishioners would come forward to speak with them, and bring them home as their own.

One too many accidents landed me in the emergency room of Boston City Hospital. I remember sitting there with my mother as I waited to be treated for a fractured elbow. I cringed as the man next to me bled through his bandages, and leaned over and whispered to my mother, "I could never be a doctor. I don't like to see people hurt." Yet that experience, followed by a summer job as an orderly in a surgical ward, solidified my resolve to become a doctor. In spite of my somewhat spotty high school record, I was admitted to Tufts College in 1926 as a premedical student.

In those days, you could enter medical school with only two years of college preparation, providing you took all the required courses, namely, physics, chemistry, biology, English, history, and a foreign language. There were about

120 students in my pre-medical class, and we were told at the outset that only thirty would make it to medical school. It was a real struggle, because in addition to my heavy course load I worked nights and summers to help pay the $300 tuition bill. In spite of this hectic schedule, I was one of the thirty accepted into Tufts Medical School, Class of 1932.

The curriculum at Tufts Medical School was of the classical variety with emphasis on anatomy, physiology, and pathology. These subjects were taught lecture-style, though the anatomy lectures were enhanced with the use of some well-worn cadavers. In my third year of medical school I was able to give up my job as a tour bus driver and took a job working as a house officer at two local hospitals. St. Mary's Infant Asylum was where unwed mothers were sent to deliver their babies. Right next to St. Mary's was St. Margaret's, where the private patients delivered their babies. Though the hospitals were right next to each other, they were worlds apart. My job was to deliver and help care for the babies at St. Mary's and help administer gas and ether anesthesia for the private patients at St. Margaret's. The $5.00 I received for assisting with each delivery was a windfall, and more than made up for the frequent, middle-of-the-night calls.

Kings County Hospital

After graduating from medical school in 1932 I applied for and got what was considered an excellent appointment for internship at Kings County Hospital in Brooklyn, New York, a 2,000-bed hospital affiliated with the Long Island

Medical School. In lieu of salary I received a white uniform, room and board.

Times were tough in Brooklyn. The economic situation was a disaster, prohibition was in full swing and provided all sorts of opportunities for graft and corruption. Irish, Jewish, and Italian gangs concentrated their activities in Brooklyn, and gangsters killed each other off at an alarming rate. My first month of work at Kings County I was required to ride the ambulance and work in the admitting department of the emergency room. This was a particularly gruesome experience. The gangs were violent and without mercy. It was not uncommon to hear a car come careening up to the entrance, brakes squealing as the driver slowed the car just enough to allow the other gang members to dump yet another body off onto the sidewalk. Sometimes we could save these victims, more often we could not. For someone who professed not to like blood much, I saw more than my share of it during my tenure at Kings County.

My appointment was for two years and was a rotating one, which meant I took basic surgery, medical, and obstetrics but could also select from other fields. I chose a month of pediatrics and neurology, and found neurology especially interesting because of the wealth of clinical material. There was a great deal of tertiary syphilis, including cases of tabes dorsalis and general paresis. The Neurology Department also took care of alcoholism in all its forms. There were the immediate concerns of caring for seizures, comas, neuropathies and dementia, as well as ongoing care for the many pathetic chronic alcoholics. Most of them were men and included doctors, clergymen, businessmen, husbands and fathers in an endless procession of misery. I often wondered why we labored so hard to help these desperately ill people, while they, most with otherwise healthy bodies, continued to soak their brains in alcohol.

I remember one patient, handsome and clean-cut, who was an anesthesiologist from a famous New York hospital. No friend or relative would have anything to do with him, and when the time came for his discharge he had only a pair of ragged trousers to wear home. I couldn't let him leave like that, so I gave him the only other suit I had. It was well-worn but clean, and I completed the ensemble with all the extra shirts, socks, and undergarments I could spare. A few days following his discharge, two police officers came to the House Officer Quarters looking for William C. Moloney. I acknowledged that was my name and they said they had arrested a fellow for breaking and entering. This fellow had shirts and handkerchiefs with the name "William C. Moloney" sewn on them. The officers wanted to take me in for questioning, but I began to laugh and explained how I had given the fellow some of my old clothes. Since the shirts and handkerchiefs had to go to the hospital laundry, my name had been sewn inside them. They departed without further comment.

The advantage of a rotating internship is that it gives a student the opportunity to try his hand at all types of medicine. It is as much a winnowing-out process as it is a learning one. I quickly learned surgery was not my destiny. My few experiences with surgical cases turned out rather badly. One early morning I delivered a baby and had to do an episiotomy to facilitate the birth. When I got through sewing up the wound, I stood up, only to find to my intense embarrassment that I had sewn my rubber glove to the girl's perineum. Another time I circumcised an infant only to have the baby's mother return several weeks later with a surprising demonstration. "Look doctor," she said. "Every time my baby pees, he pees right over his head." Sure enough, he did. I hastily arranged for a senior surgeon to repair the damaged organ and never again attempted a surgical procedure.

In spite of this, I did excel in other areas. While a medical student I had been much impressed and influenced by Dr. William Dameshek, a distinguished hematologist. As my training at Kings County proceeded I began to take particular interest in blood disorders. There was a ward at Kings County that contained sixteen patients bed-ridden with the neurological complications of pernicious anemia. These patients had acquired the disease before Minot and Murphy announced the discovery of the effectiveness of liver therapy in 1926. Seeing these patients gave me insight into the terrible neurological complications of the disease, and solidified my interest in diseases of the blood.

I completed my internship in 1934 and was offered a senior residency. I wanted to continue my training, but it was not possible on the $100 per month salary they were offering. Not seeing any alternatives, I returned to Boston to open up a general practice and move in with Josephine O'Brien, the young woman I'd met at a party my second year of medical school and secretly married in 1933, during my internship.

General Practice

The Depression was in full swing. No one had any money, and certainly not fledgling physicians just starting out in

practice. Jo and I sent out our belated wedding announcement, purposefully undated, and rented a first floor
five-room apartment in a two-decker on South Street in
Jamaica Plain. We purchased "on time" enough furniture
for a bedroom, kitchen, and waiting room (which also
doubled as our sitting room). I had a telephone installed
and began the process of setting up my practice. This was
long before the days of 911 emergency service. Back then
the telephone operators served as the conduits for all kinds
of information, emergency and otherwise. I called the local
telephone exchange and informed the operator-in-charge
that I was a new physician and would welcome receiving
emergency calls. She was receptive to my offer, and promised to put me on the list.

I next went to introduce myself to the local physicians.
I called on Josephine's long-time family doctor first. It was
not an auspicious beginning to my career. He said that it
would be a mistake for me to open a practice in this
neighborhood, and before showing me to the door, warned
me not to try and take over any of his insurance cases. The
next doctor I saw was even more peculiar. A stout man
who gave the impression of someone who didn't get up
out of his chair very often, he lived alone in a huge house.
He only charged $1.00 for an office visit, rather than the
usual $2.00, and was known in the neighborhood for his
willingness to give out prescriptions. Our meeting was
brief, as it was clear we had different ideas about what it
meant to practice medicine.

I was discouraged by these first visits, but struggled on.
I next went to a large, elegant house occupied by a much
more genial older man. He had the benign appearance of

a *Saturday Evening Post* doctor, and had a very successful general practice as well as several banking and real estate ventures. He had graduated from Yale University Medical School and enjoyed a very good reputation in the neighborhood. He assured me that he would refer cases to me, especially on Wednesdays, his day off. (I later found out that this was the day he visited a local racetrack.) I came away gratified and encouraged.

Close to my neighborhood was the Faulkner Hospital in West Roxbury. This was an outstanding hospital, with a staff made up of physicians and surgeons chiefly connected with first-class teaching hospitals such as Massachusetts General and Peter Bent Brigham. I applied for admission to the Faulkner staff, but there was a waiting period of several months, and approval was contingent upon membership in the Massachusetts Medical Society as well as the American Medical Association. I was not yet a member of either.

My practice began to take off once I began receiving emergency calls via the telephone operator. These calls were for the most part late at night and involved accidents in the home and alcohol-related events. Hardly anyone paid the $3.00 I charged for these house visits, but what I lacked in income I certainly made up for in the variety of experiences I had and the number of friendships I made.

One day, I was asked to visit a lady who had spilled a whole pot of chicken soup in her lap. The rather extensive second degree burns to her lower abdomen and groin required my returning several times to dress the burns, and I got to know her and the other members of her family. Any time I came to make a call, the grand lady would insist

I stop in the kitchen for tea and a piece of cake. This was an old Jamaica Plain family and they referred many patients to me.

Another time, I received a call to visit a family who lived not far from my office. I was met at the door by Helen Rafferty, a friendly young lady who told me her husband had had a severe cough with fever for several days. The husband was a tall, handsome Irishman who was racked with a nonproductive cough. I examined him and found scattered rales throughout both lungs. I sent him to the Faulkner Hospital for a chest X-ray. The next afternoon, I received the horrible news that his lungs were filled with golf ball-sized tumors. I went back to the house and questioned the husband and wife more carefully. They told me that five years earlier a mole had been removed from the middle of his back by a well-known surgeon. The surgeon had told them that it was a melanoma, but that he'd removed it completely. About three years later, some enlarged glands developed in the young man's left armpit. These were removed by the same surgeon and he again assured them that all the disease had been removed.

The couple had been engaged but delayed their marriage during this difficult time. When I met them they'd just been married a year. Malignant melanoma is one of the most aggressive and untreatable of all malignancies; there was nothing to be done for the man beyond prescribing increasingly larger doses of narcotics. Mercifully, he died within a few weeks. Helen was disconsolate and came to see me about his insurance papers. I inquired as to what her plans were for the future. Since she had been taking a WPA course in secretarial work, I asked if she would like to work a few days a week managing my office and doing some simple laboratory tests such as urinalysis and blood counts. She readily consented and worked for me for over thirty years. Helen was a very kind person and since my office and small laboratory were in the house, she became like a cherished aunt to Jo and my children.

I experienced some comic episodes as well as these tragic ones. One day I received a call to go to an apartment in nearby Hyde Park. When I got to the third floor an elderly gentleman told me his wife had become unconscious in the bath tub. I saw an elderly lady (she was seventy-six years-old), semi-conscious, floating in the deep old-fashioned tub. I put a sheet over her and, try as I might, I was unable to pull her out of that bathtub. She was quite well-nourished and I couldn't get a grip on her soapy, slippery skin. Her husband came to lend a hand but even in tandem we could not get her out. At last, he said, "We need more help. I will call Mother." This he did and a sprightly old lady shuffled in to assist. Between the three of us yanking and pulling we managed to get the patient out of the tub and on to the floor. Her pulse was about twenty, but full and strong and, while I was no cardiologist, I realized she had Stokes Adams Syndrome, a condition in which there is a heart block and the patient lapses into unconsciousness.

The three of us again worked in tandem to get the patient into bed, then I rushed off to my office and looked up Stokes Adams Syndrome. I found the treatment was to administer atropine sulfate, which I carried in my bag. I rushed back to the patient and administered the medication and her pulse rate became normal and she rapidly improved. When all the excitement quieted down, I inquired as to the age of Mother, our able assistant. Mother was ninety-nine years-old.

Another time I received a call to go to a basement apartment consisting of a bedroom, kitchen, and sitting room. It was an especially cold December, and I arrived to find a tiny infant in a crib, literally blue with the cold. There was no heat in the house and the child had simply frozen to death.

On yet another occasion I made a house call to the Brown family in Roxbury. They lived in an apartment over a store and were obviously very poor. Tom Brown had a job as a watchman in a meat packing plant and at an abattoir in Brighton. There were six children and the two youngest were twins about six weeks old. Both had whooping cough and were desperately ill. One infant was having convulsions along with paroxysms of coughing. Just that week I had read a letter in the *Journal of the American Medical Association* in which a doctor described how he cured an infant who was convulsing uncontrollably by injecting ether and mineral oil rectally. I had a well supplied doctors bag (next to my microscope, my most-prized possession) which contained ether and a rectal tube. The Browns had olive oil and I injected the ether and oil mixture by syringe via the rectal tube. Sure enough, the infant stopped coughing and fell asleep. Meanwhile, on examining the other twin, I found she had bilateral pneumonia. We had no antibiotics in those days and she subsequently went downhill and died, while the other twin survived.

Making these middle-of-the-night house visits was not without risk. Once I visited an Irishman, a motor man, who lived with some relatives on the third floor of a triple-decker. The poor fellow had Pick's Disease, a condition in which fluid collects in the chest and abdomen. An eminent internist was his doctor. He asked me to see this man and remove the fluid from his chest to spare him an admission to the hospital. With the patient was a very nice Irish lady whom I recognized as a nurse at St. Margaret's Hospital. They were to be married when he recovered.

I finished the chest tap and started to leave when there was a tremendous rumpus in the front room. The nurse was in the grasp of a huge and obviously intoxicated man who was attempting to throw her out of the window. I put down my doctor's bag, went over and remonstrated with him. He released the nurse and took a round-house swing at me which, if it had landed, would have knocked me unconscious. With great presence of mind I ducked, and then followed a scene out of a Mack Sennett comedy. The nurse ran downstairs and called the police while I threw chairs and other objects in the man's path as I sped from one room to the other. Finally, seeing my chance, I flew out the door, down the stairs, and out on the street. There, I met several police officers and one of them informed me that the fellow was well known to them. He had just been released from the State Insane Asylum and was crazy as well as drunk. I was happy to let the officers lead the way back into the house. I provided only moral support (from a safe distance), as they cornered him with a mattress and handcuffed him.

It should be obvious to you by now that practicing medicine brought me in contact with a wide variety of people. Just a few days after being chased and swung at, I received an urgent call to come perform a complete check-up on Cardinal Eugenio Pacelli, who was visiting Boston at the time. The pope had become ill, and Pacelli was rumored to be in line to take his place. It was critical Pacelli have a complete medical exam to ensure his good health. I'm not sure why I was the one called, but suspect it was because I was one of only a few Catholic doctors practicing medicine in Boston. I knew who Pacelli was, and I was nervous about examining him. Somehow, even standing there in his long johns, collar and funny turned-up shoes, the man had presence. I removed the bottles from my little cigar box and immediately spilled the contents of one of them. This accomplished two things: it took the shine right off the fancy mahogany desk, and made me even more nervous. I used a large needle, as was my habit, to take a blood sample from the Cardinal's ear.

As it turned out, the Cardinal had particularly meaty earlobes, and using a needle that size was akin to cutting him. And yes, I can verify, Cardinals do bleed—profusely—to the point that blood splattered all over his collar. "I'm hurt, I'm hurt," he cried out. I said a few placating words, then finished the exam as quickly as I could and backed out of there, hoping to put the whole incident behind me. I didn't think too much more about it, until I opened up *Time* magazine and saw a picture which had been taken later that same day. Apparently the Cardinal had not had time to change his collar, and my handiwork (though fortunately not my name), was visible for all to see.

These are just some of the highlights of the many interesting encounters I had during the early days of my general practice. While my income was meager, and there

were times Jo and I could hardly afford to put gasoline in
the car, I always realized how valuable those years were.
There was a certain intimacy in going into people's homes
and sharing a cup of tea with family members. It was an
enriching experience which made me feel I was doing some
good. It gave me a perspective on patient care many
specialists never developed.

Carney Hospital

In addition to developing my general practice I was especially anxious to begin a teaching career. Since I was not
yet qualified to be put on the staff at the Faulkner Hospital,
I joined the Carney Hospital in South Boston. The Carney
was also a teaching hospital for Tufts Medical School, and
I was appointed assistant instructor in medicine, teaching
physical diagnosis to second-year medical students.

The hospital was founded in 1864 by an Irish immigrant,
Andrew Carney, and was operated by the Sisters of Charity
of Montreal, a noted nursing order of nuns. This hospital
took care of the hoards of Irish immigrants who poured
into the U.S. during the days of heavy immigration. Many
of the so-called "coffin ships" came through the port of
Boston. While many died during the passage, others survived only to die once they arrived here. Many of the Irish
who did survive settled in South Boston and East Boston,
and the Carney became their local hospital. The Harvard
Medical School furnished the staff of the Carney, and the
physicians and surgeons who worked here were known to
be among the best in Boston. However, in 1913, the Peter
Bent Brigham Hospital opened its doors in Roxbury, right

next to the new buildings of Harvard Medical School, and most of the Carney staff members moved there.

The mostly poor and uneducated Irish who immigrated to the U.S. proceeded to better themselves during the latter part of the nineteenth century. Great emphasis was placed on obtaining an education. At first, jobs as policemen, firemen, and construction workers were goals. But as their economic status improved and Catholic schools and colleges were built, more and more Irish went on to professions such as law, medicine and business. However, education was largely parochial and Catholic schools, even the colleges, tended to stress classical and religious subjects; scientific subjects were not strongly emphasised. When those of Irish extraction did go into medicine, they tended to choose the fields of surgery or obstetrics. There were exceptions, but few went into academic medicine or scientific fields. The unfortunate result was a dearth of experienced, upper-level Catholic doctors.

In addition to instructing at Tufts Medical School, I was also assigned to the Carney Hospital Outpatient Department. The outpatient department was the lowest rung on a very tall ladder. Hierarchy was very strict, and it was usual to spend years as an outpatient physician before advancing to the house staff. I was strictly there to help on the front lines. I cared for patients as they came in, but was not permitted follow-up visits and could not admit any patients of my own.

Shortly after joining the Carney I began to see elderly patients with anemia. Some of these cases turned out to be pernicious anemia, others were cases of iron deficiency. There was no laboratory in the out-patient department so

I took the blood specimens back to my office in Jamaica Plain to do the hemoglobin and blood counts. Soon, the kindly old Sisters who ran the out-patient department allowed me to use a room to examine these patients, and gave me a place where I could keep my blood counting equipment. In spite of their support, there was little I could do for the patients. Other than liver extract, recently developed due to the work of Minot and Murphy, and iron by mouth, there were no therapies available for anemias. Or for most other diseases, for that matter.

The major diseases of the time were infections, most of them incurable. In *The Youngest Science*, Lewis Thomas assesses the scene: "For most of the infectious diseases on the wards of Boston City Hospital in 1937, there was nothing to be done beyond bed rest and good nursing care. Whether you survived or not depended on the natural history of the disease itself. Medicine made little or no difference." William Castle, the eminent hematologist, echoed this sentiment: "Except for conditions that could be treated surgically, our patients either recovered as a result of their own resources, or succumbed to their illnesses."

Good quality patient care, in a sterile environment, was often all I could offer my patients. Unfortunately, until I could pass the rigorous qualifications necessary for appointment to the Faulkner staff, I was forced to use several poorly run general hospitals to admit my patients, often with dire results. On one occasion I was at Forest Hills Hospital assisting the Yale-educated doctor who had so impressed me when I first called upon him. I was unaware he did surgery, and was surprised when he called me in to assist at an appendectomy. It turned out to be quite a learning experience for me, as I saw first-hand what went on behind the walls of these poorly-supervised hospitals. This doctor swiftly incised through the patient's abdominal wall, picked up the glistening peritoneal membrane with a toothed forceps and made another bold incision which cut right into the bowel below. It was a small incision, but feces squeezed out and the surgeon calmly flipped them off, wiped the area with gauze, tied a purse string suture around the wound and continued with the appendectomy. I nearly passed out, but in spite of this doctor's inexcusable performance the patient made a speedy recovery.

Not surprisingly, my relationship with this doctor turned out to be short-lived. I was covering for him during his usual Wednesday off when I was called to see one of his patients. This twelve year-old girl had been ill for a few days with what the doctor had told her parents was a sore throat. However, every time the child tried to swallow, the saliva would run out of her nose. I called the Children's Hospital and spoke to the Chief Resident. He said that it could be a case of infantile paralysis with cranial nerve involvement and to get her into the hospital right away. I arranged for her admission and a few days later she was discharged with a Thomas collar and a diagnosis of infantile paralysis. When the good doctor returned, he said I was an alarmist and that he would never refer patients to me again. He also bad-mouthed me to all the neighbors.

While terribly upsetting to me as someone just starting out, these incidents were not unusual. My experiences with these doctors and these hospitals opened my eyes to an unfortunate situation in American medicine which lasted well into the 1940s.

A Case of Bad Medicine

It was one thing to get sick in Massachusetts. It was quite another to get sick and go to a doctor for treatment. In the early part of this century, seeing a doctor was a life-risking act. There were no regulatory bodies governing the training and qualifications of physicians in Massachusetts. Anyone with a degree in medicine could take the State Board of Licensure for Medicine. Many of the applicants for the state boards were failed medical students from other schools, undertakers, nurses, or other paramedical people. The examination was entirely written, with no practical component. It could be taken repeatedly, which meant that through perseverance alone people were able to pass the exam who were not qualified to practice medicine. If you passed, you could go out and practice surgery, obstetrics, or general practice. No internship or residency training was required.

The only protection the public had from these physicians were the rules of the hospital. Unfortunately, these rules varied from hospital to hospital. Since individuals who were unqualified could not be appointed to first-rate hospitals such as the Faulkner, Carney, or St. Elizabeth's, these doctors used the smaller, poorly run general hospitals like Forest Hills, where standards were minimal or non-existent. Staff regulations at these hospitals were a joke, as I quickly learned from my Yale colleague, and so were some of the operations which took place in them. Everyone was aware of the terrible situation; it was not new.

Abraham Flexner wrote his groundbreaking report on the state of medicine in 1910. He summed up the problem nicely: "We have indeed in America medical practitioners not inferior to the best elsewhere; but there is probably no other country in the world in which there is so great a distance and so fatal a difference between the best, the average, and the worst...Conditions made uniform and thorough teaching impossible; and they utterly forbade the conscientious elimination of the incompetent and the unfit."

As early as 1885 the Massachusetts Medical Society sponsored a bill to regulate the practice of medicine. In *A Society of Physicians,* Everett Spencer said "The Society had for years been trying to enact legislation to guarantee that those who practiced medicine had the education, skill and knowledge to do so." This proposal, and a similar one proposed in 1925, was met with indifference. Dr. Edward A. Knowlton, a member of the Board of Registration in Medicine at the time, gave a paper addressing the problems of medical licensure in Massachusetts, stressing the need to update the medical practice act:

> Our medical practice act compels us to take for examination any person who is graduated from a high school or its equivalent, who has received a degree of M.D. or its equivalent from any incorporated or legally chartered school. Practically, we have to admit for examination anybody who has a degree in medicine, irrespective of the school from which the applicant comes. And they seem to come to Massachusetts in hordes from all over the world.

All medical schools operated under charters from the Great and General Court (the Legislature) of Massachusetts. These charters could only be revoked by a vote of the Legislature. So, in spite of ongoing efforts to abolish these schools, a small minority of legislators, supported by a large group of Middlesex and College of Physicians and Surgeons graduates, were able to block enactment of laws which would force them to close their doors. From 1931–1935 there were 2,003 applicants for the state board exams. 59% of those applicants failed the exam. Of those failures, 9% came from schools approved by the Society, 91% came from non-approved schools.

Massachusetts did have an outstanding institution in Harvard Medical School. Flexner descibes Harvard as having "abundant clinical material," and gives special kudos to the laboratories as "unexcelled in equipment and organization, in respect to both teaching and research." At the time, Massachusetts also had excellent medical schools associated with Tufts College and Boston University, but these institutions were more than counterbalanced by sub par medical schools: The College of Physicians and Surgeons school and the Middlesex Medical School. Flexner describes the facilities of Physicians and Surgeons as "wretched, ill-lighted, dingy and poorly equipped so-called laboratories. The clinical resources are dubious." These schools were nothing more than diploma mills; the education was terrible and practical training almost non-existent. Unfortunately, because of the loose structure of the laws for practicing medicine at the time, graduates of these schools managed to practice their own form of medicine.

That meant that Harvard-educated physicians set up practice in the same towns and the same neighborhoods as those educated at the diploma mills. Flexner underscored the risk taken by unknowing patients: "The early patients of the rapidly-made doctors must have played an unduly large part in their practical training; at whose and at what cost, one shudders to reflect."

Fortunately, throughout the U.S. stricter laws regarding certification and practice of medicine were being implemented. National Board Examinations came to be instituted and, in the late 1930s, specialty boards in medicine, surgery, obstetrical, and other fields were established. In 1936 Governor Curley signed chapter 247, a law establishing an approving authority for medical schools. This act was not effective until 1941. And it wasn't until the end of the 1940s that the last of the diploma mills literally ceased operation.

Chapter Two

CIGAR BOX
HEMATOLOGY

1935–1942

I WAS NEVER much of a cook. Whenever Jo found me at the kitchen stove, mixing up another concoction, she had good reason to be alarmed. The Carney had meager laboratory facilities, so the kitchen at home pinch-hit as a lab for my research in coagulation and bleeding disorders. I'd mix up batches of animal brains on the burners of the stove and store leftover animal body parts in the refrigerator. This worked well enough until the morning Jo opened the refrigerator door to be greeted by an exploding cow's stomach. That was the day that particular lab of mine closed for good.

By the 1930s, medicine in the U.S. had improved. New anesthesia techniques had been developed, blood transfusion perfected, and anti-bacterial substances and antibiotics were discovered. As science became an integral part of the practice of medicine, institutions such as Johns Hopkins and Harvard established higher standards for medical school admission and education. All was in place for the medical revolution that would soon occur.

Proud Day

I was accepted on the staff of the Faulkner Hospital in 1935 and this proved to be one of the best breaks of my career. The staff of the Faulkner was made up of distinguished physicians and surgeons from the faculties of Harvard, Tufts, and Boston University Medical Schools. Most also served on the staffs of the prestigious hospitals, such as the Massachusetts General, the Peter Bent Brigham and the New England Medical Center. There were frequent staff rounds and lectures. The Pathology and Radiology Departments were outstanding and the nursing services superb. Strict rules governed the activities of all staff members. Records were scrupulously kept, all deaths were reviewed by a staff committee and, if mistakes or errors of judgment occurred, the physician could be, and often was, dropped from the staff. The whole environment was dedicated to the highest quality of patient care and teaching. It was a great day for me when I was admitted to the staff.

The Rh Factor

From 1934 to 1938, two very important events occurred which dramatically advanced hematology. Alexander Weiner, a former pupil of Karl Landsteiner, discovered a new red blood cell factor in Rhesus monkeys. Fifteen percent of humans had this factor and 85% did not. Another physician, Philip Levine, also a former pupil of Land-steiner, concluded that hemolytic transfusion reactions were due to incompatibilities of the Rh-factor. If a patient *without* the Rh factor (Rh negative) received a transfusion from someone *with* the Rh factor (Rh positive), an antibody was induced that was capable of causing destruction of the Rh-positive cells. Levine also concluded that, during pregnancy, Rh positive cells from the fetus passed through the placenta into the maternal circulation. If the mother were Rh negative, she would form an anti-Rh antibody which, on passing through the placenta, would hemolyze or destroy the Rh positive cells of the infant and result in its death. This remarkable discovery explained the cause of hemolytic disease of the newborn. It was also observed that Rh-negative mothers became increasingly sensitized with each pregnancy. The problem was especially pronounced in Catholic hospitals, where multiple pregnancies were common.

Seeing the obvious need, I set up Rh typing and detection facilities in both the Carney and St. Margaret's Hospitals. The Rh tests quickly became routine, though I occasionally encountered problems I could not solve. Alexander Weiner studied one such case at my request and found an explanation for the problem. Weiner and I published an article on the case in *The American Journal of Clinical Pathology*. This turned out to be an incredible coup for me; the association with Weiner really helped propel my career. About the same time as the Rh discovery, a Danish research worker, Henrick Dam discovered that if newborn chicks were deprived of fats in their diet they developed a deficiency of a factor he named the Koagulation vitamin, vitamin K. He found that this lack of vitamin

K led to deficiency of prothrombin, which is an essential part of the blood clotting process.

Coumadin

In a seemingly unrelated event in America, veterinarians were puzzling over a bleeding disorder which was observed when cattle were dehorned. Astute investigators found that the disorder occurred only in cattle that had eaten spoiled sweet clover. Further studies revealed that the spoiled sweet clover contained a chemical substance known as coumadin. When coumadin was administered to animals, it caused a vitamin K deficiency followed by a coagulation defect evidenced by abnormal bleeding. In other words, coumadin inhibited vitamin K, and thus interfered with the production of prothrombin.

Both these findings were widely publicized in the medical literature and gave new life to the field of hematology. As Maxwell Wintrobe stated, "The introduction of new blood clotting techniques seems to have been the turning point that awakened investigators from the lethargy that existed as the result of the universal acceptance of the classic theory of clotting." These discoveries led to concrete, effective treatments for diseases that previously had been fatal. In a medical landscape best described as dismal, these events were a light on the horizon, and showed how research could be applied to achieve real results. As doctors, we began to see instances where our knowledge, and not just the patient's inner resources, could be used to heal. It was the beginning of a change in the medical mindset that would have dramatic impact in the coming years.

An immediate benefit of the apparently disparate findings of Weiner and Dam was the discovery of the cause of the hemorrhagic disorder that often accompanies severe jaundice. Many investigators had worked on the problem, and a physician pharmacologist named Armand Quick made a crucial connection. He theorized that excessive bleeding in jaundiced patients was the result of the lack of bile salts in the gastric intestinal tract. The lack of bile salts prevented absorption of fat-soluble Vitamin K. We now knew from Dam that a lack of vitamin K meant a prothrombin deficiency, hence impairment of coagulation. Finally, here was a direct explanation for the fatal bleeding that could occur when operating on jaundiced patients. Quick devised a simple laboratory test for measuring prothrombin time. This "Quick Test" was a simple, life-saving method for determining, preoperatively, whether or not a patient was lacking Vitamin K.

The Quick Test was an easy one to adminster. Plasma from the patient was introduced into a small glass tube containing calcium. When thromboplastin was added, a visible white film formed and the appearance was timed with a stopwatch. A longer than normal prothrombin time indicated a lack of Vitamin K and a deficiency of pro-thrombin. For those patients found to have this deficiency, it was a simple matter to administer the crucial vitamin.

I knew there would be a demand for this test in hospitals throughout the area, so I made up my own reagents into a Quick Test kit. Commercial thromboplastin, the key ingredient for administering the test, was expensive and difficult to obtain. However, Tom Brown, that grateful patient from my early general practice days, worked in a meat-packing plant in nearby Brighton. Tom supplied me, and later my residents and fellows at Boston City Hospital, with all sorts of brain specimens which we used in the place of commercial thromboplastin.

With ingredients in hand, I hit the road, my entire lab in an old cigar box at my side, secured with an elastic band. The tests I could perform using the contents of that box were increasingly in demand by surgeons throughout Massachusetts. In those days, there were limited non-invasive methods of making a diagnosis preoperatively, and surgical exploration was often necessary. When surgeons encountered patients with jaundice, I was called in to perform the Quick Test preoperatively. Vitamin K had been made available commercially and, if the patient proved to be Vitamin K deficient, the vitamin could be administered by injection to restore the prothrombin level. Administering this simple Quick Test could and often did mean the difference between life and death.

A much less frequent disorder, hemorrhagic disease of the newborn also was recognized to be due to a vitamin K deficiency. Again, preparations of vitamin K were soon made available and could be given to pregnant women to prevent this once-fatal disease. One day in 1938 George Allan, my former roommate and colleague from Kings County, called me for a consultation. He had just delivered a baby who was convulsing and bleeding from the nose, mouth and into the skin. I rushed to George's practice in Norwood and agreed with his diagnosis of hemorrhagic disease of the newborn. I told George about vitamin K, and he was anxious to give it a try. At that time, vitamin

K was not available commercially, but I knew two investigators at the Thorndike Memorial Laboratory who were working on manufacturing it. I lost no time in telling Dr. Robert Kark about the case. He said that he and his associate, Dr. Souter, had prepared a batch of vitamin K from leafy vegetables and would give me some to use on this infant. I dashed down to the Boston City Hospital, procured the material in a home-made vial, and returned to Norwood Hospital. The infant was oozing blood, barely alive. I put the home-made vitamin K into a syringe and injected it into the infant's buttocks. The baby stopped bleeding and eventually recovered completely. Whether the crude vitamin K did the trick or not, I never knew. However, I smile to myself when I realize the barriers of red tape and all the obstacles which would be raised today if one tried such an unscientific procedure.

Anemia

At the Carney I had begun to encounter patients in the outpatient department with anemia. Since there were no laboratory facilities there, I carried with me my improvised kit containing glass slides, pipettes, and blood diluting fluids. I would bring the specimens back to my office in Jamaica Plain, do the blood counts and look at the blood smears and the next day enter the results in the patient's chart. My work gained increasing recognition and I started to receive consultation requests from many hospitals in and around Boston. I went all over, to Worcester, Springfield, Providence, and other New England towns and cities. My chief aid was my trusty bone marrow needle. I would have

it sterilized at each location before obtaining specimens of
marrow cells. I would study the microscope slides back in
my office then call in the diagnosis. In those days there
were several famous hematologists in Boston, but none
would make visits to hospitals other than their own, and
certainly not to private homes as I frequently did.

An Office of My Own

I began to enjoy a more lucrative practice from these
consultations. In 1938 I opened an office at 39 Bay State
Road in Boston's prestigious Back Bay district. The building was located with its back to the Charles River and had
once been a very luxurious apartment building. However,
as times became more difficult, these buildings were made
over into medical offices. I ordinarily would not have been
able to afford this sort of office, but the owner, a former
dentist of my mother, was fond of me and took great pride
in my medical career. He gave me a whole suite of beautiful
rooms on the third floor for a mere pittance. This generosity allowed me to give up general practice and specialize
in hematology.

The new discoveries concerning vitamin K and the
development of the Quick Test came at a most opportune
time in my career. When I graduated from medical school,
very few opportunities existed for obtaining further graduate training in medicine, and especially in hematology. At
that time hematology was not even a recognized subspe-
cialty. My practice developed along with the specialty. And
it was not always easy going.

Cases at the Carney—Blood and Other

The Carney staff was not at all supportive of my activities. The older doctors considered me suspect, and went out of their way to ridicule me. The Chief would point me out to the students as I walked about the wards with the oversized copper water bath necessary for my prothrombin studies. "He's nuts," he'd say. He tried very hard to keep me in the out-patient department, and objected strenuously when the senior staff surgeons and obstetricians insisted I be promoted to the in-patient staff.

My life at the Carney improved dramatically with the appointment of a new Chief of Medicine. Norman Welch was a well-trained internist and a real gentleman who gave me every encouragement. With Dr. Welch's help, I organized medical staff meetings and invited outside physicians, specialists in their fields, to come out to the Carney and give talks. I printed up notices of these meetings, often at my own expense. I remember having Dr. Dameshek, a world famous hematologist, come to give an evening lecture which only five doctors attended. I was embarrassed, but Dr. Dameshek laughed it off and encouraged me to keep trying.

While we were making great headway with anemias and some of the other blood diseases, we were still helpless in the face of leukemia. I could usually make the diagnosis, but there was literally nothing to offer in the way of treatment; my presence was mostly for moral support.

One group of cases was particularly pathetic. Over a period of twelve months I saw three young adults whose cases epitomized the futility of trying to deal with acute leukemia at that time in the history of medicine. All three had similar histories, namely severe pain in the lower jaw thought to be due to abscessed teeth. In all three cases, teeth had been extracted and severe bleeding with necrosis of the gums with ulceration developed. All three were severely anemic and in the peripheral blood smears, there were numerous leukemic blast cells. Other than narcotics for their intense pain and blood transfusions, nothing could be done for these patients. At the time, there were no antibiotics nor were antileukemic agents available.

These cases came in quick succession and made quite an impression on me. I wrote an article entitled, "Oral Lesions in Leukemia" and this, my second paper, was published in *The New England Journal of Medicine.* In it, I pointed out that dentists and physicians should be aware of the possibility of leukemia in the presence of oral lesions in patients who were anemic or had purpura or bleeding gums.

Chapter Three

A "PATHOLOGIST"
GOES TO WAR

November 1942 to December 1945

IT WAS A typical fall morning: cold and wet. I was in
the rec hall, which also served as our mess hall, eating my
powdered eggs, coffee and bread. Three young aviators
came in. Two were recovering from leg and arm injuries,
the third was apparently blind. They settled themselves,
then the blind chap suddenly rose and felt his way along
the wall until he came to the end of the hall where there
was an old, battered piano. He groped his way to it, sat
down and played a few chords, then broke into the mel-
ody "As Time Goes By." In the midst of the song he
burst into great sobs. His friends guided him out into the
cold, misty morning, leaving me there to mourn his lost
youth.

In the months prior to the Japanese attack on Pearl
Harbor, most Americans watched events unfolding in
Europe with little comprehension and not much interest. Jo
and I were no different. The United States was just barely

recovering from the Depression and we were all focusing our thoughts on making a living. That all changed after December 8, 1941. As I was in the habit of doing, that Sunday morning I turned on the radio. Since Jo was at the Faulkner Hospital giving birth to Tommy, our fourth child, I was alone when I heard the news about the bombing of Pearl Harbor. My first thoughts were ones of eagerness; I couldn't wait to get over there and fight. I rushed to the Faulkner in great excitement over the dastardly attack by the Japanese. Jo, still groggy following Tommy's delivery, was understandably more concerned with her beautiful new son.

In the Army

Overnight, we went from a nation barely cognizant of European events to one gripped with patriotic fervor. I applied for a commission in the Navy but was turned down because of an old high school football injury to my left elbow. For the time being, I had to content myself with training medical students how to draw blood for transfusions. With conflict comes bloodshed, but strangely enough the U.S. Armed Forces did not take steps to equip themselves for the large amounts of blood they would doubtless need. The British were much more aware of the necessity for blood banks, and British physicians had developed a special glucose solution containing harmless anticoagulants which gradually extended the life span of stored blood up to three weeks. The first blood banks did not come into being in the U.S. until 1938.

In July 1942, I applied for a commission in the Air Force

and was accepted. I received orders to report to an air field in Texas but before leaving, I received new orders to report to the Army Medical Corps in Washington, DC. at the Army Medical School. This assignment came about through the influence of Dr. James O'Hare, a distinguished physician and professor at Harvard Medical School. He knew of my activities in the blood transfusion field and believed I could be of more use to the Army working on blood banking and transfusion. Dr. O'Hare made a few calls to some important people in Washington and this brought about my appointment to the Army Medical School.

Off to War, Sort of

I departed for Washington on November 11, 1942. Jo and the family saw me off at the train station. I left her with one year-old Tommy in her arms, and Patsy, Elizabeth, and Billy all clinging to her side. I can still see Jo's sorrowful face as the train pulled away. She never once complained or remonstrated with me, but I realized then that the sacrifices of war were being made not just by those of us in uniform.

On arriving in Washington, I reported to the Army Medical School Plasma Laboratory at Walter Reed Hospital. My duties were to bleed blood donors and help separate red cells and preserve plasma. It was an unfortunate belief that liquid plasma could be stored in small volumes and carried into battle areas. From their experience in desert warfare the British had long known that giving plasma to wounded men was not only inadequate, but dangerous. A man who had lost a great deal of blood might come out of shock with the infusion of plasma, but his remaining red cells would be diluted to dangerously low levels. This was especially hazardous for wounded men who then had to undergo a general anesthesia.

Fortunately, our efforts to produce large amounts of plasma were short-lived. Once methods of lyophilizing plasma were devised, large commercial companies became involved and soon vast quantities of dried plasma were made available. The plasma lab closed down but not before sending liquid plasma up to Boston to treat survivors of the Cocoanut Grove Night Club fire.

The Lawson General Hospital

One bright spot in my brief stay in Washington was to meet and work with Eugene Cronkite, a J.G. lieutenant in the Navy Medical Corp. He was a hematologist like myself and we had many common interests. Gene went on to a very distinguished career and we enjoyed a friendship that lasted a lifetime.

Just before Christmas 1942, I was ordered to report to the Lawson General Hospital in Atlanta, Georgia. This was a big training hospital, and medical personnel came there from all over the United States. I got leave to go home for Christmas, the last Christmas I would spend at home until 1945. After a joyous holiday with the family I packed up our only car and drove to Atlanta. There were soldiers hitching rides all along the road; their company made the long, lonely drive from Boston bearable.

The Lawson General Hospital was out on Peach Tree

Street and was crowded with all sorts of medical professors, associate professors and assistant professors. I was assigned to the Blood and Plasma Laboratory, headed by Major Grant Taylor. Taylor had been a pediatrician and an Assistant Dean at Duke Medical School; at Lawson he was Chief of the Clinical Laboratories. My job as a lowly assistant professor was straightforward: bleed donors and teach other people how to do so. I worked with several other army doctors and a group of nurses mostly in downtown Atlanta in the Red Cross Blood Donor Center. We broke up into teams and drove around Atlanta setting up mobile units for blood donations.

During our "off" hours on Sunday mornings, Taylor, myself, and several other fellows drove over to Emory University Medical School to observe Eugene Stead, the Chief at Grady Hospital, conduct an outstanding two-hour grand rounds. Stead was a superb teacher as well as a strict disciplinarian and his rounds were excellent. The standards in Stead's medical service were of the highest order. He had trained at the Peter Bent Brigham Hospital under Henry Christian and the famous Soma Weiss. Many of his fellows and residents had also trained there.

I also met Roy Kracke who was Chief of Hematology at Grady Hospital. He was a cordial man and he asked me to help out at the Blood Donor Center at Grady Hospital. While the work was not exciting, we did run into a problem with fainting in blood donors. I became interested in the problem and gathered together a large series of cases. Since syncope really did not concern the blood itself, I sought advice from Dr. Stead, an expert in the field. He was not only helpful, but gave me a letter of introduction to Eric

Bywaters, a noted English investigator in the field. I met
Bywaters and several other English physicians when I
arrived in England in 1943. The paper on Syncope in Blood
Donors was finally published in *The New England Journal
of Medicine* in 1946.

The American Federation for Clinical Research

In my daily practice in Boston I would not normally have
come in contact with men such as Taylor and Stead. One
way the war served to help me and, I believe, helped to
advance medicine, was by putting people together from all
different parts of the country. We exchanged ideas and the
result was fresh insight, a different perspective and renewed
enthusiasm. This kind of camaraderie and intellectual esprit
de corps was kept alive after the war by the medical
research societies.

One such society was the American Federation for Clini-
cal Research, a non-exclusive research society which had
been started in Boston by Dr. Henry Christian of the Peter
Bent Brigham Hospital. Fondly known as the Young Men's
Christian Association, and sometimes irreverently referred
to as the "Young Squirts" society, it was a young, young
Turks society. Dr. Taylor introduced me to the group and
I joined in Atlanta.

Nothing seemed to last very long in the Army, and
Grant Taylor was transferred across town to the 4th Service
Command Headquarters. Shortly thereafter, I received orders to report to Colonel Koonz's outfit at Fort McPhearson, also in Atlanta. This Colonel was "regular Army" and
an unbelievable despot. He had the good sense to gather

together some outstanding physicians, especially those expert in tropical and infectious diseases, but he had no consideration for our collective talents. In fact, he seemed to delight in showing his contempt for us. Professional men that we were, we retaliated by plotting ways we would throw him off the ship once we were sent abroad.

A Hematologist Becomes a Pathologist

My role at Fort McPherson was consulting hematologist (although I was still only a Captain) and part of my duties were to travel around Georgia and Alabama visiting prisoner-of-war camps in search of exotic diseases. The prisoners we encountered were tough, Nazi-types, many from the Afrika Corps. Their diseases, however, were not particularly interesting. Infectious hepatitis was the most exotic disease we encountered.

Since I had been assured that my unit would be staying in Atlanta for at least six months, I found a house out on Peachtree Street, near Buckhead, and sent for Jo and the children. Only Patsy was of school age and we managed to enroll her in a very good school run by Belgian nuns. But after only a few months of family life, I received orders to report to Fort Bragg, North Carolina. The Colonel would not let me go without a fight, and came with me to headquarters in Atlanta. My interview there was very brief. The Medical Administrative Corp Colonel said I was to be Chief of the Pathology Laboratory at the 347th Station Hospital, a 350-bed hospital in England. I quietly pointed out that I was a hematologist, not a pathologist. This did not carry much weight; his mind had been made up. He

responded, " You look through a microscope, don't you?"
I had to admit that I did. He then said, "Then you are a
pathologist. Dismissed!" I went home and broke the news
to Jo and the children. The next day, I helped them pack,
and some kind Southern neighbors drove them to the train.
Later, I got leave and drove the car to Boston, then
returned to Fort Bragg via train to report for duty.

Fort Bragg was a much different environment from
Lawson. We lived in wooden barracks and, since there was
no hospital or other facilities, had little to do but exercise.
I lost twenty pounds in my brief stay there. There was
daily close order drill, calisthenics, road marches, and even
practice with a carbine crawling through a simulated mine
field. This latter exercise really scared me as it made the
prospect of war, and its attendant consequences, quite real.

Off to War, Really

In early November of 1943, orders came for us to prepare
to go overseas and we were moved to a staging area in
New Jersey. We had a twenty-four hour leave. There was
a rather somber farewell party in New York which Jo
attended. A few days later our group boarded the Queen
Mary for the trip to England. With most of the 9th Air
Force on board with us, we were a prime target. The ship
zig-zagged all night, and traveled at a fast thirty-five knots.
We knew this was too fast for a submarine to catch us, but
there was always the possibility of encountering a wolf
pack. Many of us stayed up during the night worrying
about it.

The trip across the Atlantic was blessedly uneventful.

When we arrived in Scotland we were put on a train and given strict instructions to keep the blackout curtains drawn. Once we reached Oxford we were put on trucks and taken to our hospital site, which was just that, a site and nothing more. No hospital facilities had yet been set up. We were assigned in groups of six to huts no bigger than a single-car garage. The weather was dreary: cold, foggy, and generally miserable. We had a pot-bellied stove for warmth but very little fuel for it. Mitchell, one of the doctors, took it upon himself to go into town to scavenge for coal. He was promptly arrested by the village constable and taken before a judge who sternly lectured him about the sacrifices necessary in wartime. Al admitted his guilt and suggested they send him back to the States, where at least it was warmer. Of course Mitchell was released but his actions did nothing to improve our relations with the local population.

For the next few months we did nothing but drill and march. The tedium of this was relieved by calisthenics, after which we drilled and marched some more. In early spring we were moved out to the countryside into large company tents. It was still very cold and wet, but at least now we were cold and wet with a bit more room. In April the sun came out, the fog lifted and lo and behold we had been in the midst of beautiful countryside the whole time.

We moved on to the 347th Station Hospital in Marlborough. This was an old British hospital which, we were told, had taken care of casualties from the ill-fated Dieppe raid. Since the British were in short supply of building materials and plumbing supplies, the hospital was poorly constructed. But we made do with what we had and gradually I was able to organize a laboratory. I was concerned about my ability to fulfill my assignment as Chief Pathologist, but fortunately I had good junior officers on my staff: one a bacteriologist and the other a biochemist, as well as a private who had been an undertaker's assistant. A British pathologist at Radcliffe Infirmary in Oxford was very kind and offered to show me how to do an autopsy. I learned the rudiments of the procedure, and was later relieved to find out that I would not be required to tie off vessels at autopsy since there would be no embalming of the corpses.

By this time I had already been in England several months, but had yet to experience the war first-hand. That changed that day at Radcliffe Infirmary when a very young airman was brought into the morgue. While flying as a waist gunman, both his legs had been cut off by machine gun bullets and he had bled to death on the plane ride home. He looked so young and so pitiful. And I remember him particularly because he brought home to me, for the first time, the realities of war.

The Work of War

Once our hospital became operational, most of the cases we received were trivial, mostly pneumonia, hepatitis, and infectious mononucleosis. My first autopsy was on a young soldier who had been struck by a jeep, an occurrence so frequent it was known as the German secret weapon. My second autopsy was a young officer who had committed suicide with his pistol. Detailed pathology reports had to be made in these cases.

Unlike World War I, extensive epidemics of pneumonia

and meningitis were not encountered. We did see the occasional case of it, and one night a patient with cerebrospinal meningitis turned up. Our Chief of Medicine, Herbert Rathe, was an excellent internist. He wanted to treat the patient with penicillin, which had just become available. Since penicillin was still in such short supply, we were told we could not use it for this case. The precious drug was reserved for the exclusive use of treating gonococcal infections in combat troops, the rationale being that these soldiers needed to be cured quickly in order to be sent back to the Front. This policy infuriated all of us, but our hands were tied.

Nevertheless, we all knew that penicillin would soon become readily available. So to familiarize ourselves with the proper dosages, Rathe and I went to Oxford to pay a visit to the lab of Dr. Florey, the chemist who worked with Fleming to isolate penicillin. We rang the bell on a Saturday afternoon, and were greeted by an Englishman in knickerbockers. He told us he was Dr. Florey's assistant, Dr. Chain, and that Dr. Florey was in Moscow teaching the Russians about penicillin. Rathe asked Chang if he could show us how to calculate the dose of penicillin in Oxford units. Chain readily agreed and took us to his rather dingy laboratory. There, he stuck his finger with a large and rusty needle, obtained a drop of blood, and placed it on an agar plate with a number of holes punched in it. He then placed penicillin of various amounts in the holes and, by noting the size of the areas which became clarified, he could calculate the dose of penicillin.

As we prepared to leave, he offered to show us how they extracted the penicillin. He led us into a huge hall that had once been the hot house for the university's horticultural department. Here the penicillin mold was grown in large, flat, earthenware jars. After the jelly-like wart formed, it was poured into vats where it was beaten with what looked like homemade wooden paddles. The material was then poured into what Chain assured us was the distilling apparatus, but which looked all the world like a moonshiner's still. Since the British were desperately lacking supplies, this apparatus was joined together with pipes of various sizes and colors, and gave a rather grotesque, and decidedly non-scientific, appearance. The jelly-like material wended its way through pipes, tubes and tanks until, after what seemed an interminable wait, it emerged, drop by drop, into a precious collection vial. We were fascinated and a bit amused. Chain smiled and said, "I bet I know exactly what you are thinking. This reminds you of a Rube Goldberg cartoon!" He could not have been more correct. We quite expected bells and whistles to go off.

I would be reminded of this episode some months later when I attended a large gathering of medical personnel in London. The first speaker was an American Colonel, a specialist in genito-urinary infections, who presented his findings on the treatment of sulfa-resistant gonococcal infection in 350 U.S. soldiers. All infections had cleared up speedily and his paper was greeted with great applause. The moderator of the meeting was the famous Sir Henry Dale. He congratulated the speaker, then asked if the discoverer of penicillin had anything to add to the discussion. At which point Dr. Fleming, a rather unimposing man dressed in simple civilian clothes, got up and proceeded to the podium. He congratulated the speaker on his findings and said, with some lament in his voice, "I have only been able to procure enough penicillin to treat three cases of sulfa-resistant gonorrhea." Then he couldn't help but add, "But then it's appropriate the Americans have all the penicillin, since they're the ones with all the gonorrhea."

Unnecessary Losses

A station hospital does not have a large staff and at times duties were doubled up. I was in charge of the laboratories, and also nominally in charge of the Officers Ward. We had very few patients, and just a few days prior to D-Day the wards were entirely empty. Just before we were moved out, two WAC sergeants were admitted to the empty ward for treatment of advanced gonorrhea. One afternoon, the nurse in charge carried two blue envelopes to each of these girls. These envelopes were each filled with one gram of sul-fadiazine, the standard treatment at the time for gonorrhea. The nurse had removed these envelopes from a large cardboard box in which all such envelopes had been stored. These were the last two envelopes in this particular box. The WACs did as instructed and quickly drank down the powder with a glass of water. The nurse went back to her station and on reaching the end of the ward, was horrified to hear strangled cries coming from their room. In the time it took her to run the length of the ward, both women were dead. This caused great consternation and an imme-diate investigation took place.

I heard nothing further about it until a few days later, when I was visiting Smith's Book Shop in Marlborough. As I was browsing the shelves, two U.S. Army MPs came up to me and asked if I was Captain Moloney. When I acknowledged that I was, they saluted and said firmly, "Captain, please get in the jeep." I mildly remonstrated but they were large fellows and very business-like. Realizing I had no choice, I got into the jeep and was driven back to the hospital at breakneck speed. There, I was ushered into a rather dark room in a barrack-like building and told to sit down. No one offered any explanation and I didn't have any idea what was happening. Soon I was ushered into another room filled with officers, some of high rank. I was directed to the witness stand of what I now realized must be my court marshall, and told to raise my right arm and take the oath.

A major in the Adjutant General's office then began to question me about the incident with the WACs on the Officers Ward. He pointed out that I had signed out all the narcotic orders and was responsible for everything in the Officers Ward. I acknowledged that this was so but stated that it was a formality and a routine practice. This did not please the examining officer, but after a few more questions I was dismissed without any explanation. That evening our Colonel came into my hut and told me that I was completely on my own, that he would not be assuming any responsibility for the deaths.

Through no fault of my own, this could have been the end of my medical career. But since preparations for D-Day were occupying everyone's attention, the matter was not pursued further. Later, I found out from my sergeant that the culprit, an American sergeant in the medical corps, had been found and arrested. He had been using his position as hospital pharmacist to peddle drugs. His practice

was to hide his supply of cocaine in the little blue sul-
fadiazine envelopes, then tuck them away in the back of
the supply box. The fellow went on leave, no doubt thinking the cocaine was safely hidden. By an unlucky coincidence all the sulfa drugs were used and only the two
envelopes containing the cocaine remained. These were the
envelopes given to the two WACS. I never did learn what
happened to the pharmacist; the invasion took place and
everything else faded into insignificance. I have often
thought of those two women and the strange tricks of fate.

D-Day

Early on the morning of D-Day, immense flights of U.S.
and British bombers and fighters filled the skies. The skies
were cloudy and overcast but the flights continued nevertheless. At the same time, the invasion ships began to land
troops on the Normandy shore. We received fragmentary
reports over the radio of the battles that were being fought
less than 100 miles away from us. Battalion-aid men came
ashore with the combat troops, and a short time later
Mobile Army Surgical Hospital (MASH) units also landed.
These MASH units consisted of young general surgeons,
anesthesiologists, and surgical technicians. They did a mar-
velous job operating, while under direct fire, on abdominal
and chest wounds which would have been fatal unless
immediately treated.

Intense efforts were made to evacuate the wounded by
employing Landing Ship Tanks (LSTs) or any available
ships. On arriving in England, the wounded were quickly
moved directly to Evacuation Hospitals equipped with

plenty of whole blood and staffed with skillful surgeons and nurses. But as the troops pushed farther inland our hospital began to receive large numbers of badly wounded men. We were an intermediary point between the Front and the Evacuation Hospitals, and our job was to separate and triage the various types of wounds, transfuse the men, then send them along to an Evacuation Hospital. The wounds we saw were horrendous, especially those from high-explosive shells. Abdominal, chest, and head wounds were common, as were missing limbs and compound fractures. All came to us enclosed in bulky, blood-stained casts. I took two sergeants, each with a hospital cart filled up with bottles of whole blood, and we proceeded down the aisles. I would say "Give this fellow four units," or, "give that one six units." There was no time to type or crossmatch; we gave every soldier "O" blood.

Large company-sized tents were set up to accommodate the overflow from our barrack-like hospital. Severe winds made the tents noisy and unstable, and it was difficult to take care of patients. Fortunately, the townspeople responded magnificently to the emergency; they bathed and cleaned up the wounded, gave them fluids and food, and were of tremendous help. After about twenty-four hours of straight work, I gave in to my exhaustion. I stepped out of the tent, sat down, and wept from sheer frustration. I pulled myself together, took a brief nap and went back to work.

As I resumed what seemed like an endless procession of plasma and blood transfusions, I heard a gasp behind me and turned to see a young soldier in a body cast go into violent convulsions. Before I could get to him, he was dead.

I figured he'd had a pulmonary embolism, and continued on to the next soldier. This soldier had a similar convulsion and also died very quickly. Shaken, I took a close look at the plasma bottle and noted fibrous clots floating in it. I opened the bottle and the distinct odor of perfume emerged. Since I had worked in the plasma laboratory at the Walter Reed Hospital, I knew something about plasma. I also noted the label on the plasma bottle: the Benvenue Perfume Co. The perfume company had received a government contract to produce dry lyophilized plasma. However, all the liquid had not been removed properly from the bottles, and the plasma did not go entirely into solution. I went immediately to the Colonel and reported the situation. He impounded all the suspected plasma and I sent a jeep to a nearby General Hospital to get a fresh supply prepared by a well-known manufacturer. We used the new plasma without further incident.

The next morning I got a summons to the Colonel's office. I was met by an angry Major, pacing back and forth. He immediately began upbraiding me, accusing me of being an alarmist and a troublemaker. I stood my ground and told him it would be criminal to use any of the Benvenue Perfume Company plasma. The Major stalked out and my Colonel said, "Moloney, I hope you are right." Within forty-eight hours, numerous reports poured into London concerning fatal reactions from the use of this plasma.

It is difficult to recreate the horror of that summer. The first flood of wounded was overwhelming. The soldiers were all thirsty, dirty, hungry, and in pain. I tried to describe it to Jo in one of my many letters home, but couldn't bring myself to mail the letter to her. I kept the letter for myself, as a record of where I'd been and what I'd seen, and as a reminder of all those soldiers, as young as they were brave, who passed before me.

6/21/1944, England

Dearest Jo:

I have had a chance for a few hours to sit down, so I am going to write to you first, take a shower and go to bed. We opened for air evacuated casualties a few days ago, it seems ages now. It will live in my mind as the worst whirlpool of human misery and suffering I have ever known. I guess perhaps I am a little depressed tonight and very tired. Not a healthy sort of fatigue but a nervous, jittery sort of tiredness. Hope I can sleep tonight. Of course, opening up as we have in a make-piece hospital, conditions have been far from ideal. But none of us realized what we were getting into, I am sure. When you think you have worked to the limit, and everyone else has too, and then you are forced into the appalling necessity of looking forward to more than you have already done in that rush, well it is depressing. However, we are much better organized and I am getting some system worked out for my blood transfusion work.

We have used incredible amounts of blood and plasma and I am simply amazed that men live that have such extraordinary injuries. It is grotesque, the impact of it at first leaves you aghast, then I think you get numb and insensible to all but some things which break through your shell. A smile on a young face that should have been sorrowful, a few tears trickling down when a fellow wakes up to find a hand or a leg gone–the pathos of those little things penetrates where the impact of some horrible wound makes your senses recoil and harden.

We filled our buildings and had patients in tents, the wind howled and tore at the canvas, it was like aboard a ship with the rocking and creaking of the piles and ropes. The noise of the wind drowned out some of the cries of the wounded. Looking into these places, filled and pulsating with pain and suffering, one wondered if a sudden miracle has opened the gates of Hell and its fury was revealed for a brief view.

The wounded talk of battles, soldiers talk of being "pinned down," the terror of the accurate Heine 88 mortar —"they could put them in your pocket." "I saw the bastard in a tree, he was camouflaged very well but I got four slugs into him." "We didn't use our B.A.R. guns, they spotted us too quick, and bang, a mortar shell." "Those damn bazookas tore the top off the tank, top gunner just blew up in little pieces," etc, etc.

But most lay silently in pain, or groan softly, "Please Captain, fix this cast?" "Please move my leg?" "Can't you do something for me sir?" And the million things to do, all thirsty, most ravenously hungry after several days of meager or no food. Ward boys and nurses worked until they nearly dropped from exhaustion.

Throughout the months of July and August we continued to receive large numbers of casualties. We would make emergency adjustments to casts and dressings then send the patient along. Wounded were transferred by ambulance to various hospitals, but since there were not enough ambulances to meet demand, buses were pressed into service. It was a rather macabre sight to see these large Army buses filled with its strange cargo of bandaged soldiers, peering out.

I described the routine of daily life in a journal entry made August 28, 1944:

"It is good to get back. Today I feel good. Tired yesterday evening. The queue of ambulances was long, about fifteen ambulances plus a day, but with ambulatory patients. It is a pretty incongruous sight. One sees a huge sightseeing bus packed with these poor chaps, pale and wan faces peering out, heads turbaned and bandages and arms in casts and slings. Many in battle dress, some in pajamas. It looks for all the world like a nightmare sightseeing tour that has just come through the valley of death.

The wards filled up rapidly, a forest of frames with sprouting ropes and apparatus and the grotesque shapes of large casts. Pain-racked forms hidden by the covering of the bed. The inevitable casts! Blood-soaked and cumbersome, all bearing the inscription of the date of wounding and nature of the injury. "W.I.A. F.C.S. H.E. debridement 25/7/44" etc. All the necessary data, label of pain and inscription so impersonal! What nights of agonized sleeplessness you prescribe! You pale and bearded boys with your foxhole dirt still on you, aged youths, matured by pain and terror. Where is the glory and the adventure of battle? Enemy unseen, a mechanical and impersonal shell, tearing and renting flesh and bone. In the midst of all this suffering, one can only draw from it the fortitude and courage with which these terrible wounds are borne.

Few break down. At least, thank God, it lies in our province to relieve pain! To make them clean, to feed them and make them comfortable becomes of primary importance. As they go back the shock and psychic trauma of their experiences, the gaping flesh and shattered bones, will lose its raw edge. Immobilized by their ugly yet so necessary plaster casts, bolstered by blood and plasma, protected by penicillin and sulfa drugs, they begin to heal. Many will need more surgery, more manipulation and alignment of broken bones, some will lose hands or parts of them. But all the skill and all the modern advances of surgery and medicine will be at their disposal. One feels that as they go back, they go back for further good care and better chance to recovery and restore to normal living."

Prior to D-Day I cannot say I felt particularly connected to the war. I went through my routine blood work, keeping supplies typed and stocked. After D-Day, after seeing how badly the blood was needed, after seeing first-hand how giving the correct blood could be the difference between life and death, I never again considered my work a waste of time.

One morning, I was rounding up some walking wounded when I noted that one GI was missing. I called out his name and found him in a dimly-lit bathroom, trying to shave. He was very young and walked slowly, bent over, to his bunk. I looked at his W.I.A. tag and saw that he had been wounded in the chest. He took off his shirt and I noted a healed, round bullet wound just to one side of his heart. Posteriorly, there was a large healed wound of exit. I wondered how he had survived such a wound and, after examining him, concluded that he must now have a large blood clot in his left pleural cavity. He told me that he was with the 101st Airborne Division and had parachuted on

D-Day plus two hours. Their mission was to seal off areas so that the rest of the division could land. However, the Germans were waiting for them and while he was taking off his parachute, a German soldier came up close and shot him at point blank range. He said he got up and started to run, then added, "You know, Captain, bubbles of blood kept pouring from the wound and I finally collapsed."

When he came to, he was surrounded by a group of very tough looking SS troops. He was sure they were going to kill him but an older man, apparently not a combat soldier, pleaded with them to spare his life. So, they made a litter and carried him to a German field hospital. The older man told the young soldier that he had once worked in Brooklyn. When the Americans overran the field hospital some days later, this boy was evacuated and arrived in our hands. His only regret about the incident was that he never got a single shot off.

General Patton's Armoured Division

Sometime in August 1945 General Patton's 7th Armoured Division came through Marlborough and temporarily took over our hospital for their headquarters. It was very impressive when Patton went by. Enlisted men got out from under vehicles they were working on just to salute the officers. It was all very G.I.

When we were finally able to reclaim the facility, we decided to host a dance for all the doctors, nurses and hospital personnel. This turned out to be a bad idea. Just as the dancing began a crowd of tough armoured division officers, all of them tank commanders, came charging in.

Fights immediately broke out, and our limited security forces were badly beaten up. The ringleader was a nasty Italian Major. He was vicious. My days making house calls in Jamaica Plain prepared me for this. I knew exactly what to do. I beat a hasty retreat. After calling the nearest M.P. post, I was distressed to see a short while later a jeep arrive with one lone man. He was a Colonel, large and bulky, but he didn't seem much of a match for the swaggering Italian. I held my breath and watched from a safe distance. He got out of the jeep and calmly asked the wiseguy to return to his outfit. In response, the Major reached over and pulled the Colonel's cap down over his ears. Without missing a beat, the Colonel then picked the fellow up, whirled him around, slam-dunked him into the rear of the jeep and drove off with him. Nothing came of the matter; as it turned out, the Major was a good tank commander.

I took no satisfaction in seeing these same troublemakers again several weeks later. As Patton's troops moved inland, we received our usual miserable quota of casualties, second-hand from the MASH and evacuation hospitals. Among them were those same brash young warriors, many of them now with limbs off and great healing wounds.

Rh or CDE?

In September I was ordered to report to the 162nd General Hospital as Chief of Laboratory. Attendant with the move was a promotion to Major. This gave me an increase in pay and allowances and was of some help to Jo at home. The hospital was located in Arrington, about six miles from Cambridge. It was near a huge airfield which had been a major airbase for the 8th Air Force. The 8th Air Force had seen a great deal of action and had sustained heavy casualties; it was being replaced by elements of the 9th Air Force. We served as their base hospital, but by this time the large bomber commands were operating from air fields in France. Our hospital was being prepared to receive mostly orthopedic cases and was staffed by excellent general surgeons and orthopedic specialists. Of course, a great deal of blood would be required and I was kept busy ensuring the blood banks were kept full. I made some particularly good friends here, especially Major David Sprong, a Johns Hopkins trained surgeon of outstanding ability.

While we were in the process of getting our laboratory and other facilities organized, a B-17 on a practice run crashed one night in a nearby woods. Four of the crew men were killed outright, six survived, five of them badly injured. They were taken to our hospital, but I had no blood to give them. I rushed in a jeep to the Addenbrooks Hospital in Cambridge. There, I was greeted by a friendly civilian doctor who told me he was Dr. George Taylor. I told him of our problem and he immediately gave me all the type O blood they had in their Blood Bank. I rushed back to Arrington but in spite of the transfusions, all five of the injured airmen died. Incredibly, one crew member survived uninjured.

The next morning, I drove back to Cambridge with the empty blood bottles. The British were desperately short of all medical supplies and I knew they would want to reuse those bottles. We were lavishly supplied with equipment, and our careless treatment of our supplies stood in stark contrast to the care the English took with their meager belongings.

Dr. Taylor was a distinguished scientist who worked with R.R. Race, Robin Coombs, and others who had been bombed out of London and were installed in the Cavandish Laboratory in Cambridge University. There they typed the blood of all the Royal Navy and Royal Air Force personnel. Since they did not have enough centrifuges for the blood typing, they set up wooden blocks with holes bored in them. They placed A serum in a small tube in the first hole. In the second hole they placed anti-B serum. In tubes three and four, they put the patient serum and added to tube three, A cells, and to tube four, B cells. In the fifth tube they carried out the Rh typing. Since they did not have enough centrifuges, they let the tubes settle while they had tea. The tubes would then be shaken and the results read. These tests were very accurate, and compared to the sloppy methods of blood typing in our laboratories, their method was a revelation. Many of the laboratories in the U.S. Army were run by pathologists who had little or no experience in clinical pathology. There was little interest in hematology, and our blood was often mistyped.

George Taylor took me to Race's laboratory and introduced me to Race and his staff. The staff proved to be a very bright group of young ladies; his chief assistant was Ruth Sanger, a very pretty and friendly Australian lady. Race and his associates were particularly interested in the genetics of blood groups, and were undertaking to study the Rh and other subgroups.

With the expanding use of blood transfusions, more difficulties were encountered with transfusion reactions within the ABO system. George Taylor and R.R. Race had been interested in the genetic aspects of red cells and, since they were engaged at Cambridge University in blood typing for the Royal Navy and Air Force, they had ample blood specimens to study. At the same time, Weiner and his associates in the U.S. were investigating the Rh subgroups. This gave rise to a bitter debate between two schools of thought: Race wanted to name the new factor CDE, carrying on from the A and B antigens, while Weiner preferred the Rh nomenclature. Actually, the problem was much more profound and involved the concept of paired genes (CCDDEE) versus Weiner's belief that there was only one locus for the Rh factors. The CDE system was easier to understand and to teach but in the long run Weiner's concept proved to be correct.

Race gave me a very cool greeting, then asked me what kind of a person was Alexander Weiner. When I told Race that I was not well acquainted with Weiner, he challenged me. "You were a co-author on his latest paper," he said. I acknowledged that this was so, but explained that it was a case report, and that I'd never really worked directly with Weiner. Race then took a letter from his pocket and asked me to read it, which I did. It was a very arrogant and insulting letter in which Weiner forbade Race to publish any more of what Weiner called "his foolishness." All I could do was tell Race that Weiner did have some unpleasant characteristics which made him disliked by many people. Weiner should have received the Nobel Prize, but he so antagonized people he was never awarded it.

In spite of this inauspicious beginning, R.R. Race, Taylor and I became friends. Taylor and I would take bicycle rides together, I upon Taylor's daughter's bike. After the first ride, Taylor said, "Moloney, you do not need to call me 'Doctor Taylor.' In this country we say 'Taylor' among friends." I found it a great tribute; he was a fine person and an outstanding scientist.

On one of my visits, Taylor introduced me to a young, good-looking fellow named Robin Coombs. Coombs was a veterinary immunologist who worked in a laboratory above Race's. Taylor said to me "Coombs has an interesting test he wishes to show you." Whereupon Coombs mixed up some red cells in an albumen suspension, added serum to be tested, and the red cells rapidly and visibly agglutinated. Coombs had reasoned that anti-Rh antibodies did not necessarily exist only in the serum but could be fastened on the surface of red cells. However, the cells would not clump if placed in saline solutions; if albumin or serum were added, visible agglutination took place. This was the justly famous Coombs test. It was an epochal discovery which proved to be particularly important in Rh problems, and an invaluable addition to our techniques for detecting so-called "incomplete antibodies."

In the spring of 1945 I received a letter from John Spellman, a doctor with whom I had become close during my early days at the Faulkner Hospital. His son, John Jr., had been wounded in the Battle of the Bulge. In spite of the fact that his brother, Cardinal Francis Spellman, was Vicar for all the Armed Forces, the family had not been able to locate the son, nor did they have any accurate information on the nature of his injuries. John Jr. had been in a protected unit, posted to Washington, D.C.. However, when it was decided to form a 3rd Army and mount an invasion from Southern France, new formations were rapidly created and men from reserve and special service units were sent over to France. Most of these troops were not combat trained and they were sent to an area believed to be quiet—the Ardennes.

One morning, young Spellman's outfit was hastily summoned to move out of their barracks and get into troop carriers. John was last out of the barracks, and as he sprinted for the troop carrier a shell from a Tiger Tank hit it, killing all his fellow soldiers. John laid unconscious for a full day before being discovered. He was evacuated to England and eventually turned up in a hospital in Wales. I got leave and went by train across England and managed to see young John and talk to his doctors. I was able to write back and reassure John Sr. that while his son was badly shell-shocked, doctors felt convinced he would fully recover.

The summer of 1945 passed and with it the war. I was still awaiting discharge when I got word in October that Jo had been admitted to the Faulkner Hospital with a severe uterine hemorrhage and had undergone a hysterectomy. The Red Cross arranged for me to get compassionate leave and I flew home. It was a joyful reunion, although my boys were disappointed because I had not killed any Japanese.

Chapter Four

HEMATOLOGY ON THE HOME FRONT

1945–1952

MY GROUP was caught up in the surge of excitement surrounding new discoveries. Money was tight at BCH, but that did not dampen our eagerness to participate. I paid $68.00 from my own pocket for a water bath to use to study hemophilia. In those days, the water bath was the chief tool for studying bleeding problems; it was there we measured the clotting time of the blood specimens set in the 37°C water. In light of the discoveries we were able to make, that $68.00 now seems like a small price to have paid.

The years following my discharge from the Army were the most important ones of my career. It was during this time that I established my reputation as a hematologist and laid the foundation for the research I would later do with the Atomic Bomb Casualty Commission. Not surprisingly, this period was also one of the busiest times of my life.

I was officially discharged from the Army in December, 1945 and with the help of Helen Rafferty re-established my

practice at Bay State Road. I also rejoined the staff of the
Faulkner and Carney Hospitals. And at the request of Dr.
William Dameshek, I became an instructor in laboratory
medicine at Tufts Medical School.

I was stretched thin. My consulting practice had me
running hither and yon seeing patients at the more than
thirty hospitals that dotted the New England landscape.
Some days I would visit three different hospitals, and rarely
were they close to one another. In general I had excellent
relations with the staffs at these hospitals, but problems
arose at the Carney and St. Elizabeth's.

Cardinal Rules

It was common knowledge that St. Elizabeth's, like the
Carney, lacked distinction. Over the years, the staff had
become inbred and content with practicing below standard.
My old friend John Spellman, a distinguished surgeon, was
now Chief of Surgery there. I knew John was aware of
the problems at St. E.'s, because he and I had often discussed them. Since St. Elizabeth's Hospital was owned by
the Boston Diocese, it was directly under the control of
the Archbishop. Possibly because Spellman's brother was a
Cardinal in New York, the Archbishop relied heavily on
John for guidance. I felt that with the combination of the
Archbishop's ear and the Cardinal's influence, Spellman
could accomplish great things at St. Elizabeth's.

When John asked if I would be Chief of Medicine, I
gave it careful thought. All my professional life I hoped a
Catholic hospital would emerge with an excellent, well-
trained staff and take its place among the nation's best

hospitals. It seemed to me that if the Beth Israel Hospital, representing the best in the Jewish community, could reach such high levels of excellence, why not a Catholic hospital? I began to think that as Chief of Medicine at St. Elizabeth's, I would finally have my chance to fulfill my vision of creating a world-class Catholic hospital.

Both the Carney and St. E.s were used by Tufts Medical School for 3rd and 4th year teaching. I could not be on staff at both hospitals; I had to make a choice. The Chief of Medicine at the Carney, Dr. Norman Welch, was a fine physician and a good friend. He urged me to play a more active role at the Carney, but I had already offended many of the older members of the staff and neither they nor I were happy about the prospect of my career continuing there. In December 1945, after meeting with the doctors of St. Elizabeth's, I told John I'd accept the position of Chief of Medicine.

With acceptance, however, does not come approval. While John's persuasive talents worked on me, they did not work with the in-bred crowd of St. Elizabeth's. Catholic doctors working in Catholic hospitals made up a small, close-knit community in those days. I had made a reputation for myself at the Carney Hospital, and no doubt word of my rebellious activities had made its way to St. Elizabeths. The staff probably feared for the safety of their own jobs. If they did, they were right to do so. My appointment was passed over in favor of a member of the staff. In a spirit of cooperation, I called to congratulate him and said I would be glad to help with organizing staff meetings and other activities. There was an ominous silence, then he said coolly, "If I need any help from you, I will ask for it!" The phone went down with a bang, and I knew that was the end of my career at St. Elizabeth's. The Irish Mafia had cooked my goose.

Curing the Incurables

John was not particularly bothered by this set-back, and asked me to take a look at another ailing Catholic hospital, the Holy Ghost Hospital for Incurables. Given my track record this seemed a bit like asking me to hammer the nails into my own coffin, but out of friendship for John, and a genuine desire to elevate the standard of medicine in these hospitals, I once again agreed to help.

The Holy Ghost Hospital was a fifty-year-old institution run by the Sisters of Charity from Montreal. These Sisters had a great reputation for bedside nursing, and the hospital was immaculate and well-run. But an inspection by the Massachusetts Division of Health found the medical education sub-standard, and the two-year course for Licensed Practical Nurses (LPNs) was ordered shut down until medical staff could be upgraded and laboratory and X-ray facilities installed. John asked me to do my own assessment of the hospital. During my visit I met a gracious Sister Superior, Director of Nursing Schools for the Order in Montreal. She also had been asked to survey the situation, and together we toured the halls. We were aghast at conditions. In the course of my assessment I found one pernicious anemia patient going without treatment, and another in a corner who had lapsed into a diabetic coma, apparently unnoticed. Most of the cases I saw that day were crippling arthritis, strokes and other neurological disorders.

The fifty beds reserved for terminal cancer were mostly empty.

Most of the patients were at the Holy Ghost as a last resort, and were sent to us from the prestigious general hospitals such as Boston City, the Peter Bent Brigham and the Massachusetts General. It was sort of a holding place for chronically or terminally ill patients. There were 300 beds at Holy Ghost; 250 of them were reserved for patients with chronic diseases, and the remaining fifty beds were for terminally ill cancer patients. The staff physicians were a group of twelve elderly men, each of whom served on a rotating basis for a term of one month. Their duties consisted of visiting patients each morning, writing prescriptions and transferring patients in distress to whichever local hospital had room for them. Since there were no diagnostic laboratory facilities and no X-ray equipment, there was little else these doctors could do for the patients, even if they *had* been so inclined. And any inclinations they did have ceased mid-afternoon. Thus, the hospital was without an on-staff physician after 5:00 every evening, night, holiday and weekend.

Following my visit, I made a number of suggestions. A new medical staff was essential, with specialists in surgery, internal medicine and neurology. Also a laboratory facility and an X-ray department. Equally imperative was obtaining fourth year medical students to work as house officers to cover the hospital at night and on weekends. I felt lucky to find two Tufts medical students willing to take the job in exchange for room and board. I was also able to recruit several of my younger colleagues: a surgeon, a neurologist, an oncologist and an internist to join the staff. This all took place within the space of a few months during the summer of 1946. I felt we had made a good start.

However, less than a week after putting this new system in place I got a call from the medical students informing me they'd been fired. I was furious and immediately called John Spellman. After a great deal of trouble, John was able to arrange for us to meet with Archbishop Cushing. His Eminence was not happy to see us. He came striding into the meeting and growled, "What do you guys want? You're just a bunch of rich doctors driving around in fancy cars." Quietly, and with as respectful a tone as I could muster, I interjected that all of my services had been volunteer. Al Murphy, a surgeon who'd joined us at the meeting, made it clear that none of us had fancy cars. Somewhat mollified, the Archbishop confessed his dilemma with handling the hospital situation directly. "Fellows, you know these Sisters," he said. "They are women, and they're also French." Apparently he found such a concentrated dose of femininity overwhelming, but after listening to our story he promised to take action.

Within a few days several more Sisters came down from Montreal to review the situation. The Mother Superior was replaced by a simply wonderful Sister who was most accommodating. We were delighted with the change, but the group of staff doctors were outraged. They called a staff meeting, and the Archbishop, finding out about it, ordered me to go. I knew how unwelcome I would be at that meeting and my expectations proved correct. I was challenged the minute I walked in. When I told them I was there at the Archbishop's orders, they went into executive session, took a vote and resigned as a body. I had the meeting room, and the hospital, all to myself.

Fortunately, my friends and associates quickly came to my rescue and we worked together to build up an excellent staff. We adjusted the admissions requirements to increase the cancer bed population since this seemed to be the area of most urgent need. We started treatment programs using the few chemotherapy agents available at the time, primarily nitrogen mustard. Oncology was just becoming a recognized specialty and we developed a relationship with oncologists at Tufts Medical School.

I stayed on as Chief of Medicine and Hematology at the Holy Ghost Hospital. There was no salary with this position, but I did have the opportunity to meet and work with some highly skilled physicians. One of them was Dr. Shu Chu Shen. Dr. Shen had worked with William Castle at the Thorndike Memorial Laboratory and was a member of the Tufts Medical group of oncologists. He had a small laboratory space at the Holy Ghost where he ran experiments on small animals, chiefly mice and rats.

Blood Banking

One important experience I had both before and during the war was my work in the field of blood transfusion. My acquaintance with Race and Coombs made me an expert by association, and as the Rh incompatability problem made itself manifest during routine blood transfusions, consultation requests poured in. One call from St. Margaret's Hospital was to see an infant with Rh incompatibility. The infant was already jaundiced but had not yet developed any of the neurological features of kernicterus, a potentially fatal problem caused by the buildup of bilirubin in an infant's bloodstream. Dr. Louis Diamond of Children's Hospital, a pediatric hematologist and one of the pioneers in the Rh field, came out to the hospital and I assisted him in doing an exchange transfusion that saved the baby's life.

After this procedure, Dr. Diamond urged me to organize the blood banks in all the Catholic hospitals. Because the problems of Rh incompatibility become more and more pronounced with each pregnancy, Catholic women were particularly in need of this service. Since I was already consulting with many obstetricians at area hospitals, it was a natural extension of my services to help them set up blood banks. I did this at the Carney, St. Margaret's, the Faulkner, Cambridge City Hospital, and several others. I actually set up an Rh laboratory in my Bay State Road office and many of the obstetricians sent blood specimens to me to be typed. This furnished me with a very welcome source of additional income.

In spite of the interest in the Rh problem, Boston City Hospital ignored it. They had no blood bank, and seemed in no hurry to establish one. I expressed my astonishment to a close friend, a well-known member of the BCH medical staff, and the next day received a call from Dr. Martin J. English, Chairman of the Board of Trustees at BCH and a very formidable figure. Dr. English lost no time berating me for criticizing Boston City Hospital. He pointed out that BCH had the Thorndike Memorial Laboratory, home of the greatest hematologists in the world, who did not need any advice from me. I tried to explain that I shared his high regard for the Thorndike Memorial Laboratory but that the staff there was interested in anemias, not Rh problems.

I called my friend back and told him that as far as I was concerned, BCH and Martin English could go to the devil. But someone else must have brought up the possibility of legal consequences, because the very next day Dr. English again called me at my office. Without offering any apologies, he agreed to meet me at BCH to discuss the Rh problem. I showed him my lab there, which was not much more than a broom closet, then proceeded to follow him to the Mary E. Curley Children's Building. This building was comparatively new and had been named in honor of James Michael Curley's wife. He brought me up to the eighth floor, which was entirely unoccupied, and told me the space could be mine, provided I did not smoke. I boldly outlined plans for a large laboratory space, a conference room, and an office. Within six weeks we had a beautiful new laboratory facility equipped with microscopes, centrifuges, water baths, and plentiful supplies. In addition, I was provided with a technician and a laboratory helper.

About this time I received a visit from a physician who was assistant to the Chief of the Boston University Medical School Services at BCH. He had heard of my experience at St. Elizabeth's and told me he was authorized to offer me a position on the B.U. Medical Service as Clinical Professor of Medicine, and Chief of one of the two BU medical services at BCH. The combined jobs came with a part-time salary of $5,000. The money was enticing, but my loyalty was with Tufts. I had always been connected with Tufts, and had often made hematology rounds on the

Tufts Medical Services at the Boston City Hospital. The Chief of Medicine and Director of the Tufts Medical Services at BCH was Fernando Biguera, an excellent internist and cultured gentleman from Guatemala. He and I had become good friends.

I postponed a decision about BU pending a visit with Dwight O'Hara, Dean of Tufts Medical School. I told Dr. O'Hara about my offer from Boston University and he was considerably disturbed. He proceeded to outline his plans for me. At Dr. Biguria's urging, I was to be made Associate Director of the Tufts Medical Services One and Three at BCH, as well as a Clinical Professor. These positions came with a part-time salary of $5,000. I accepted Dean O'Hara's offer and the very next day began expanding the Medical School's research activities using the new Rh laboratory as a base of operation. Although the Tufts Services did a fine job in training young physicians to practice medicine, they did little clinical research.

Even though the Tufts 1st and 3rd Medical Services at BCH provided a major source of teaching beds for Tufts students, Dr. Proger, Professor of Medicine, was so preoccupied with building up the New England Medical Center that he did very little to support teaching or research at BCH. But turning the New England Medical Center into the outstanding medical center they hoped it would be was difficult. The location of the medical school and the Pratt Diagnostic Hospital were very unfavorable. Situated as they were in one of the poorer and crowded sections of Boston, there was little room for development. Nevertheless, it was here that the venerable Boston Dispensary was located. And while it was not much more than an outpatient facility, it was the nucleus around which New England Medical Center was created. Even after the Pratt Diagnostic Hospital and the first buildings of the N.E. Medical Center were erected, there were still not enough medical and surgical beds available. Thus, Tufts continued to rely on the Carney Hospital in South Boston and St. Elizabeth's Hospital in Brighton, along with several smaller institutions.

Boston City Hospital

During the late 1940s, Boston City Hospital was at its peak of fame and accomplishments. The hospital's emphasis on excellence in clinical activities and research had rightfully earned it a leading position among all the teaching hospitals in the U.S. Largely due to the presence of the renowned Thorndike Memorial Laboratory, the BCH was the first municipal hospital to provide facilities and support for research. It was there that the work of Minot and Murphy, followed by William Castle and his colleagues, created new frontiers in clinical medicine. Great clinicians in other fields, like Soma Weiss and Max Finland in infectious diseases, and Williams in endocrinology, were also on the BCH staff. Along with these outstanding individuals, neurological staff included people like Derek Denny-Brown and Houston Merritt. The famous Mallory Institute of Pathology played an integral role in the development of this superior medical institution, and an appointment to the BCH as an intern or fellow was much sought after.

Visiting physicians would make two- to three-hour rounds five days a week. In lieu of salary they received a place to park and privileges to eat in the House Officers Dining Room, which, believe me, was no privilege. The medical internship was for one year followed by a year of junior and senior residency. Of course, no salaries were paid, but room, board, and uniforms were provided. In those days, few house officers were married and reasonably good quarters were provided in the House Officers Building. Often, after the first two years of training, residents would seek specialty training elsewhere.

The Tufts Medical Services had four floors of the BCH Medical Building. Each floor consisted of a large open ward of sixteen beds, several smaller four-bed wards, and one room reserved for dying or mentally disturbed patients. There was only one common lavatory. Since the hospital population consisted chiefly of the unwashed and the unwanted, the environment was not auspicious for private patients. Visiting physicians could not, and did not, admit private patients unless under extremely desperate conditions.

Tufts had good company at BCH with both the Harvard and the Boston University Medical Services. A good deal of competition existed between the medical schools, but, by and large, the staffs got along very well. Since Harvard had the most prestige and was far better funded, they tended to have a somewhat superior attitude; for the most part, it was well earned. The subspecialties, such as infectious diseases, hematology, endocrinology, and renal diseases were chiefly run by Harvard. However, B.U. developed some outstanding people in gastroenterology and renal diseases, and Tufts provided a pulmonary service.

Masters of the House

As well as being prestigious, the Boston City Hospital was an exciting place to practice medicine. We had many interesting cases and a remarkable house staff. One of the truly outstanding young men there was Bill Harrington, a second year resident on the Tufts 3rd Medical Service. I had met Bill before I took the job at BCH. One night, about 9:30 PM, this young, fourth year medical student dressed in a soiled white uniform came into my research laboratory at the Holy Ghost Hospital. He said he was working at the nearby Cambridge City Hospital, and asked if I'd take a walk over with him to look at a bone marrow slide. Harrington had decided that the patient had multiple myeloma but the visiting physician disagreed. This put me on the spot, but I reviewed the slide and agreed with Harrington's diagnosis. I was delighted to learn later that he would be one of our interns on the Tufts Service at BCH.

Another remarkable young intern was Fred Stohlman. Fred had attended Georgetown Medical School and came from a prominent family in Washington. He was a very tall, heavy-set fellow and, like Harrington, was a tremendously hard worker with a brilliant mind. He went on to become Professor of Medicine at Tufts, and headed up the medical department at St. Elizabeth's. He died tragically in a plane crash. Upon hearing of his death, Betsy Bunn, the wife of my colleague Frank Bunn, had the instant reaction, "But he's too big to die." In every way he was larger than life.

Another person who played a major role in my life was my co-worker Jane Fay Desforges. Jane graduated from Wellesley College and Tufts Medical School, took a year of pathology, then an internship in the Third Medical Service at BCH. After a junior residency, she proceeded to Salt Lake City and spent a year in hematology with Max Wintrobe. She came back to BCH as Chief Resident on the Tufts Medical Services. Jane was outstanding and soon became involved with Bill, Fred, and myself in a variety of projects. Jane was greatly interested in red cell problems, and being of an analytical mind, she delved into the rapidly developing field of red cell enzymology.

One of the good things that did come out of World War II was the discovery of primaquine sensitivity. It turned out that when troops going to the Pacific were given primaquine for protection against malaria, ten percent of black soldiers developed hemolytic anemia. Research revealed that ten percent of blacks lacked an enzyme that protected against primaquine-induced hemolysis. This discovery started a flood of research efforts and resulted in a remarkable advance in knowledge concerning red cell enzymes. Jane also was involved with sickle cell anemia and Mediterranean anemia along with the newly discovered role of erythropoietin. Jane and her husband, Jerry, became my life-long friends. She rose to become Professor of Medicine at Tufts Medical School, an editor of *The New England Journal of Medicine*, and recipient of many honors in the field of hematology.

Of all the house officers, Bill Harrington was the most imaginative. Once he treated an elderly lady who was admitted with a severe hemorrhagic disorder. The first consultant that saw her was from the Thorndike Memorial Laboratory and he had carried out the usual tests, including a prothrombin time (Quick Test). He found the patient had a twelve-second prothrombin test and no explanation of the cause of the bleeding was forthcoming. Bill, who had already built up a reputation among the house staff, was asked to see the patient. The Thorndike consultant had carried out the prothrombin test using a commercial rabbit brain thromboplastin. This was an expensive reagent and, in our group, we could not afford to buy the material. So Harrington obtained some human brain and produced thromboplastin for the Quick Test. However, now the prothrombin time was sixty-five seconds.

Harrington repeated the test using other human brain thromboplastin with similar results. He called me and asked if I could get my patient, Tom Brown, to procure material from various animal sources, such as sheep, pig, and steer. Harrington drove out to the abbotoir and brought the brain specimens back to the BCH. Then, working throughout the night, he made up batches of thromboplastin from the various animal brains and two other human brains. The prothrombin times with all animal brains was ten to twelve seconds, with the human brains it was over sixty seconds. Harrington reasoned that the patient had developed an auto-antibody for thromboplastin which did not react with animal brain. He published an article on his findings in the *Journal of Laboratory and Clinical Medicine* in 1950. At this time, the concept of an auto-antibody was new and controversial; Harrington was ten years ahead of his time.

The advances in our understanding of coagulation, and the new problems which were brought to light as a result of those advances, were critical to our development as clinicians, as well as to the development of the field of hematology. The fellows who worked with Jane and me developed as scientists in part through their care of patients. They were able to treat the bleeding disorders, while, at the same time, work through problems in the supportive environment of our laboratory. Each fed the other. Caring for patients and following their progress provided invaluable clinical information. That information, in turn, allowed us to learn more about the disease, and at times, conquer it.

Bleeding Disorders

In the summer of 1948, I drove to Buffalo with Harrington and several other young doctors to attend the second annual meeting of the International Society of Hematology. There I heard Paul Owren of Norway describe his research. Owren had been studying clotting disorders in both the male and female members of one Norwegian family. It was an unusual case, and he perservered throughout the German occupation of Norway in order to conduct clinical studies on them. The result was the discovery of Factor V. The classical coagulation factors, calcium fibrinogen, thrombin, and prothrombin, had been discovered more than fifty years previously. Owren's discovery was a landmark one. As Max Wintrobe has noted, the discovery of Factor V was a major accomplishment and opened up new avenues of research.

While Owren was making his discovery, F.H. Laskey Taylor and his associates at the Thorndike Memorial Laboratory, along with Professor Edwin Cohn of the Harvard Physical Chemistry Department, made discoveries of their own. Working together, they were able to separate from plasma the coagulation factor missing in hemophilia. Known as anti-hemophilica globulin (AHG), this discovery, along with the Owren's discovery of Factor V, stimulated a great deal of new research. Harrington, Stohlmann and I published several reports on the cases we encountered. Our lab rapidly became involved with a number of important problems. Since investigation of bleeding disorders was most urgent, much of our early efforts were directed to patients with hemorrhagic disorders. There was a large population of patients with cirrhosis of the liver, and hemorrhaging from esophageal varices was a dramatic event. A variety of other bleeding disorders were also encountered, and we published several reports on these cases.

The bleeding problems we saw were frequently dramatic and often life-threatening. One case was of special importance: a twenty-four year-old woman in labor had been admitted to St. Elizabeth's Hospital. Fetal heart sounds could not be heard and she was noted to have large ecchymoses, or bruises, on her body. Also, she began to bleed from the gums. The obstetrician called me and I came over to see the patient. Her abdomen was swollen with the baby, but it was also very hard to the touch. The obstetricians made the diagnosis of abruptio placenta, a condition where the placenta is torn away from the uterine wall. It is of course fatal to the infant but in rare cases a generalized coagulation defect is created in the mother and becomes a calamitous complication.

I had never seen anything like this before. I looked at her peripheral blood smear and noted the presence of platelets, which normally participate in the formulation of blood clots. I then took specimens of her venous blood to the hospital laboratory, and found that despite incubation in a water bath, the blood did not clot. I could hardly believe my eyes and, by chance, noticed some thrombin preparation in the refrigerator, used to help stop bleeding by local application. I took some thrombin and added it to the patient's whole blood and also to her plasma which I obtained by spinning down the red cells. Again, no clot occurred. Then I knew the patient had afibrinogenemia, or lack of fibrinogen. Obstetricians were well aware of this rare condition but hitherto no one was aware of deficiency of this important coagulation factor.

It happened that directly after the war, surplus supplies of plasma and plasma products became available for research. I had been selected to represent Tufts on a committee organized by Dr. Charles Janeway at the Children's Hospital to distribute plasma products. The week before this case occurred, I attended a meeting in Dr. Janeway's office and he mentioned that they had treated several children with congenital deficiency of fibrinogenopenia with injections of purified fibrinogen. Dr. Louis Diamond had been in charge of the cases of afibrinogenemia so I called him (it was now about midnight) and told him about my case.

He agreed it was a case of acquired fibrinogenopenia and then I asked if I could have some fibrinogen for the patient. He pointed out that unlike a baby, the adult would require 8 to 10 grams of fibrinogen. He had a supply of ampules, some had 0.1 grams, others had 0.5 grams, so he collected all the fibrinogen available, gave me the lot and wished me good luck. I dashed back to St. Elizabeth's Hospital where the obstetrician and a general surgeon were scrubbed up awaiting my return. I put the various lots of fibrinogen in a 50 cc syringe suspended in distilled water. I told the surgeons that as soon as the fibrinogen was administered, they should operate at once removing not only the dead fetus, but also the uterus.

By this time, the patient was unconscious and her breathing was stertorous; huge bruises had appeared all over her body and blood was oozing rapidly from her mouth. The fibrinogen solution was thick and gluey; I could barely push the plunger through the syringe. As soon as I finished the injection, I took a specimen of venous blood from the other arm vein. The blood clotted before I could withdraw the needle and I was very concerned that she might have a large clot embolism. The surgeon completed the Cesarean section and removed the soggy, hemorrhagic uterus. They put in large sutures to prevent the wound from disrupting and continued blood transfusions. Remarkably, she regained consciousness, the bleeding stopped and she continued on to full recovery, though it took days for her to clear the huge ecchymoses and subcutaneous hemorrhages. We did not know the cause of the fibrinogenopenia; my own theory was that it occurred due to release of thromboplastin from the fetus or the uterus.

In 1949, Paul Owren came to Boston to give a talk on his work with Factor V. Unfortunately, the lecture was not well publicized and was poorly attended, with the members of the Thorndike Memorial Laboratory staff notable by their absence. Bill Harrington did attend the lecture and was very upset by the lack of recognition for Owren's work. He called me after the lecture was over and told me of his dismay, adding that Owren was staying in a "flea-bag" hotel on Huntington Avenue. I got into my car and collected Paul Owren along with Bill Harrington and brought them back to my house in Jamaica Plain. I had warned Jo that we were going to have a guest and she hurried around moving children about to make room. Paul, Bill and I stayed up late that night discussing clotting problems. The next morning I got up a little late and found the esteemed Dr. Owren in the kitchen chatting with Jo and drying the breakfast dishes.

Follicle Follies

Owren's visit was a nice distraction from my ongoing trouble with finding research grants to fund the lab research. So when Frank Gardner, who had been a fellow at the Thorndike Memorial Laboratory, called and asked if I would be interested in working on an anticoagulant problem sponsored by Squibb Pharmaceutical, I was more than receptive. The project was to investigate a new heparin-like drug called Paritol, and Squibb would give me an $8,000 grant for the work. I was overjoyed and promptly enrolled Harrington and Stohlman in the project.

At the time, there was considerable interest in developing anti-coagulants, in part stimulated by the unfortunate deaths of several young athletes from pulmonary emboli following surgical procedures. Since we required only test tubes and a water bath, we were able to start the project immediately. Paritol, like heparin, had to be administered intravenously or subcutaneously; it proved to be actually somewhat more potent than heparin and the effect lasted longer. We proceeded with the study administering the drug to "high-risk" patients, i.e. those with deep vein thrombosis, pulmonary emboli, decompensated cardiac patients, and others known to be at risk for pulmonary emboli.

We had enrolled about forty patients in the study when I departed for England in 1950 to attend a meeting of the International Society for Hematology. I was gone for two weeks and when I arrived home, was greeted by a very worried Fred Stohlman. He informed me that all the patients on Paritol had become completely bald. This was most distressing and made all the more so because of the concerns of Stohlman's father, a well known trial lawyer in Washington, about the possible legal implications. I asked Fred if any people in the group were in contact with one another. He said none were, and that the nature of their diseases tended to keep them apart. I told Fred under no circumstances to let these bald men see each other. I felt pretty sure the baldness was a temporary side-effect, but nonetheless it was a disturbing one.

As it turned out, many of these patients had serious cardiac problems and some of them died. At autopsy, the discovery of hyaline-like deposition in the kidneys brought the research project to an immediate halt. The Squibb

Company kindly allowed us to keep the residual research funds but, needless to say, Paritol never made it to the commercial market.

Young Squirts Grow Up

I was disappointed to find that the Boston chapter of The American Federation for Clinical Research, the group I had joined in Atlanta, was no longer holding monthly meetings. I felt it was important for these burgeoning scientists to have an environment for sharing opinions and exchanging information, so once my lab was up to speed I called Dr. Christian to inquire about starting up the Federation again. He discouraged my involvement, saying that many of the original members had gone on to become members of the more prestigious American Society for Clinical Investigation; he didn't feel there was sufficient interest to keep the Federation going. I was discouraged, but simply could not believe this to be true. There were too many bright, energetic doctors at the Boston City Hospital. What they needed, I felt sure, was a forum for sharing information about their ideas and discoveries. I knew what a catalyst such a forum could be for generating new ideas, and I was determined not to let the Federation die.

A valuable consequence of my war experience was the connection I now had with people from many different places. Since I knew many of the people on staff at the better Boston hospitals, I called them up to see if they'd be interested in reviving the Boston chapter. The response was enthusiastic. Just as I had done in my early days at the Carney, I found some speakers, had leaflets printed up and posted them myself, then paid $15.00 to reserve a room at the Boston Medical Library. That first lecture was well-attended by people from the Thorndike and the Massachusetts General Hospital. From then on we had regular meetings. They were informational in their own right, and turned out to be something of a proving ground for doctors just starting to present their research.

We purposefully ran the meetings using the same format that was used at the annual convention of the American Society for Clinical Investigation. The speaker had exactly ten minutes to present, then five minutes for questions. Several of my fellows presented at the Federation, then went on to great success at some of the larger annual conferences. I am convinced that the emergence of this, and other, research societies did a great deal to promote scientific and academic medicine in the USA.

Road Trip

In August 1950 I took a trip to Cambridge, England to attend the third annual meeting of the International Society for Hematology. In those days one had to pay one's own way, so we went over on the old Queen Mary, steerage class, four of us to a room with a salt water shower. The meetings were held at Cambridge University and were well organized and well attended. I had two papers on the program; one with Bill Harrington on the treatment of multiple myeloma with urethane, the other on Rh sensitization in pregnancy. I met a lot of old friends, Rob Race, Ruth Sanger, Robin Coombs and Paul Owren, as well as many other people involved in Rh research, including Alexander Weiner and Philip Levine.

We had a great garden party at the home of Dr. Race's wife's family. I took some pictures with an early-model Polaroid camera. There were individual snapshots of Coombs, Race, Ruth Sanger, Paul Owren, and many others. One picture showed Weiner and Levine assembled with a group of other prominent Rh people. The prominence of the people in the photo was enough to make it remarkable. But the fact that Weiner and Levine were within a few feet of each other and still smiling made it a rare photo indeed. There still was some controversy surrounding the grouping of Rh blood, and both men harbored resentment. Some years later Philip Levine asked me for a copy of the picture, which I obligingly sent along. Imagine my surprise when it turned up in Max Wintrobe's book, *Hematology - The Blossoming of a Science,* attributed to Levine! Such is fame.

Bill Dameshek was at the conference, and he introduced me to John Kennedy and James Gavin, hematologists from Ireland. We immediately became good friends and John Kennedy, who was Chief of Pathology and later became Dean of Galway Medical School, invited me to come to Ireland to speak at the Joint Meeting of the Irish and British Medical Societies. I readily agreed to the trip and flew over in July of 1951. I stayed at the Eggerton Hotel in Salt Hill and the next day visited Galway Medical School to give my lecture. The members of the British Medical Society were there in full force along with doctors from Scotland, Northern Ireland, and of course, Irish doctors from Dublin, Cork, and Galway. My lecture on Rh sensitization in pregnancy was well received; I had put a lot of time and effort into it and it was published in the *Journal of the Irish Medical Society.*

The following day, I drove to Dublin with Kennedy and gave a talk at the Rotunda, the famous obstetrical hospital. The next evening I gave a talk at Hollis Street, the Catholic obstetrical hospital. As I should have expected, I immediately got into a difference of opinion with a pig-headed Irishman. Having been brought up on the Carney Hospital Staff, I gave as good as I got. It was a memorable trip.

After the meeting, I flew on to Oslo where I visited Paul Owren and made rounds at the Rikshospitalet. Then on to Rome where, through John Spellman's brother, Cardinal Spellman, I was granted a private audience with Pope Pius X, the former Cardinal Eugenio Parelli. I hoped it would not involve bloodshed, as had occurred in our first encounter during my early days at the Boston City Hospital. If the Pope remembered, he had the good grace not to mention it (or to run screaming from the room).

After seeing the Pope, I went to Paris and visited Professor Eyquem at the Pasteur Institute. He was involved with the Rh problem and introduced me to a young man named Michel St. Paul who wished to come to the U.S. to work with me. We made the arrangements and Michel followed me to Boston to work with me at Boston City. Michel turned out to be an outstanding young man, very much interested in immunological problems. We were able to obtain a few animal cages in the Surgical Research Laboratory at BCH and Michel and I experimented on immunizing dogs to human lymphocytes obtained from patients with chronic lymphatic leukemia. We did manage to produce an antibody which was active in fairly high titre, and we carried out various absorption experiments. I submitted a paper to *Nature* which was turned down on what I felt were rather flimsy grounds. Michel did publish a paper, in French, on blood groups in dogs and an abstract of a paper on the antigenic properties of human leukocytes.

From Paris I proceeded to Northampton and boarded the old Queen Elizabeth for the trip home. One of my cabin mates was a young man going to New York on a medical fellowship, Jerry James. We became good friends and Jerry lent me $10.00 to help ease my passage home. Jerry was engaged to Sheila Sherlock who was already a famous pathologist. Later on, Sheila and Jerry came to visit me in Jamaica Plain and Jo was somewhat nervous about meeting someone so distinguished. Well, Sheila came in the door, shook hands with Jo, and said "Do you mind if I take off my shoes? My feet are killing me!" So much for formality.

About this time I received a letter from John Kennedy, asking me to employ a young Irish doctor named Stephen Shea. Stephen's father was Professor of Anatomy and former Dean of the Galway Medical School. Stephen was a "brain" and had a fellowship that paid his way. By this time, the Rh laboratory was getting pretty crowded, but we continued to carry out various research projects. Stephen Shea was a genuine intellectual but he was not at all interested in clinical medicine. He became a faculty member in the Pathology Department at the Mallory Institute and several years later transferred to Yale Medical School.

Bill Harrington continued to do outstanding work and

Fernando Biguria and I went to see Sam Proger about the possibility of keeping him on with us. We had heard of a rather generous fellowship that was to be awarded to an individual on the Tufts Medical Services. However, Dr. Proger had no interest in us and the award was given to one of *his* fellows. I was livid. Here was one more example of BCH getting no support from Tufts. We were poor second-cousins to the grand New England Medical Center they were trying so hard to create. Bill was offered a fellowship in St. Louis and went on to an outstanding career in hematology. Fred Stohlman also left us for the United States Public Health Service, where he worked under the direction of George Brecker, who was one of the outstanding researchers in the field of cell proliferation. Fred teamed up with George Brecker and Gene Cronkite, and the three of them embarked on a remarkable series of accomplishments involving bone marrow stem cells and control of hematopoiesis. This trio produced some of the most important work on cellular proliferation in recent history.

Practice, Practice, Practice

My private practice continue to escalate. Since I was now publishing papers in the prestigious medical journals, I became the doctor to call whenever there was a difficult case. As a result, I saw a lot of interesting ones, and some of the patients really touched my heart. One young couple had been college sweethearts and were engaged to be married. I had the difficult job of telling the woman she had acute leukemia. In spite of my dire predictions for her longevity, they married anyway. She died just a few months after their honeymoon.

There were many cases like this, and the outcomes were all the same. As my patient population grew I saw more and more die of leukemia. Just as I never became accustomed to seeing blood, nothing ever eased the pain of seeing so many young people die. The treatment available at the time was hopeless in the face of leukemia. At best, we could put patients into remission, but none of them lived even as long as a year.

Boston Doctor Cures Leukemia

One memorable patient did survive. I'd been called down to a small hospital in Rhode Island to see a young soldier, just back from the war. He'd already been diagnosed with acute leukemia. I was called in primarily to support the diagnosis, and administer any additional help I could. With a somewhat heavy heart I entered this dark house. The curtains were drawn and only a few lights were on. The patient sat upright in bed, and even in the dim light I noticed right away that his color was unusually good for someone with leukemia. I did the blood counts. Sure enough, his white counts were sky high, but not from leukemia. I had the delightful job of telling the young man that he was suffering from mononucleosis. A simple course of antibiotics put him right, and earned me the distinction of a headline in the Rhode Island papers the next day: "Boston Doctor Cures Leukemia."

Would that it were so. The reality was that all of the leukemia patients I saw quickly died. Driven by the simple desire to see my patients survive, leukemia became my main area of interest. Unfortunately, I didn't feel my interests were much supported. Tufts was still focused on establishing the New England Medical Center, and I saw no future for myself at the Boston City Hospital. I continued to scurry from hospital to hospital, but in many cases my efforts were to no avail. I was becoming increasingly frustrated and disillusioned, while running myself ragged in the process. I was seeing so many patients that I was in a fair way of becoming rich, but it was at a price. I'd come home nights exhausted and stagger through the door. And in spite of working so hard, I didn't feel as though I was making progress in my career.

Propitiously, I received a letter from Grant Taylor, my old friend from Atlanta, who was now stationed in Hiroshima, Japan as Director of the Atomic Bomb Casualty Commission. They were beginning to see cases of leukemia among both the Hiroshima and the Nagasaki survivors, yet there was no one stationed out there who knew anything about leukemia. "It's your duty to come out here as Director of Research," he told me in no uncertain terms. I saw this as a lifeline and grabbed the opportunity. Here, finally, was my chance to make a real difference. By studying cases of leukemia in its early stages, I felt sure I could make some seminal discoveries. I discussed the opportunity with Jo, told her of my increasing unhappiness at BCH and with Tufts, and she said, "When do we go?"

I was amazed. Here we were with four children, two of them teenagers, and she never hesitated. "Where you go, we go," she said. Three months later, we were on our way.

Chapter Five

MY TROUBLES
WITH RADIATION

1952–1954

WE WERE MET by Grant Taylor and taken to our house in Nijimura, a village about twenty miles from Hiroshima on the inland sea. Nijimura was a new development, built by Australian occupation forces, and had the distinction of being the site of the airfield from which the Japanese kamikaze pilots took off for the carriers en route to Pearl Harbor. This bit of trivia was not uppermost in our minds upon arrival. What *was* rather pressing was the almost overwhelming stench coming from a wood pulp factory across the inlet from the house. The factory was closed on most days, but just happened to be up and running the day we arrived. It was not an auspicious welcome.

The atomic age began with the dropping of the atomic bombs on Hiroshima and Nagasaki in August 1945. Shortly after Japan's surrender, the United States sent in a joint Army-Navy commission to assess the damage. They recommended a program be established to study the long-term biological and medical effects of the bomb. President Truman sent up a Committee on Atomic Casualties, and from that, a field organization called the Atomic Bomb Casualty Commission (ABCC) was established in Hiroshima and in Nagasaki. The objectives of the ABCC were to identify and study survivors for somatic (bodily) effects and for genetic damage. Special efforts were made to evaluate the effect of radiation on the growth and development of children.

Laboratories were opened up in each city and formal observations began in 1947. The cities had been practically wiped out, so there were many obstacles to overcome. All sanitary and other public health services had been destroyed. There were shortages of everything, and medical supplies were no exception. There were no antibiotics, bandages or even sterile dressings. The Japanese government's response to the catastrophe was almost non-existent.

With an assist from the Navy, supplies were brought in and buildings erected in Hiroshima. In Nagasaki, intact buildings were occupied and cooperation with surviving members of the medical faculty was established. Actually, there was surprisingly little hostility from the defeated Japanese. Many doctors, nurses and technicians eagerly joined the ABCC staff.

The ABCC was funded by the Atomic Energy Commission, but actually was controlled by three separate groups. It's a well-known fact that you can't run a committee with three heads. What further exacerbated the complicated bureaucracy was the fact that all three committees operated from Washington. Few of the decision makers had even seen the ABCC first-hand, yet they had the power to dictate policy from 7,000 miles away. I didn't realize it prior to accepting the position of Director of the Adult Medical Program, but this structure would turn out to be a real stumbling block.

Once Jo and I made the commitment to go to Hiroshima, we didn't look back. Understandably, there was a flurry of activity prior to our departure. In addition to the logistics of packing up a household, we also had to fly to Washington D.C. to get our State Department visas. In those days, Japan was an occupied country, and you needed either state department visas or military orders to go there. We got our visas, along with official traveling orders and inoculations, and left in March 1952.

We were excited about the adventure, but had our concerns. Our son Billy was fifteen years-old and our daughter Pat thirteen; we worried how they would adjust. In addition, we'd heard news of high incidences of cholera and polio in Hiroshima, none of which boded well for four year-old Tommy.

Trains, Planes, Slides and Dinghies: the Long Journey to Japan

We took a train from Boston to L.A., where we boarded a Pan Am Clipper which was to take us the rest of the way to our new home. For the first hours of the trip all went well, then I looked out the window and saw that one of the four propellers had stopped. We were several hours into the flight, right in the middle of the ocean, and I knew we were beyond the point of no return. Taking the only course of action that occurred to me at the time, I went up to the bar in the front of the plane for a drink. I waited rather fearfully for the next move, while at the same time trying to appear unconcerned. Shortly thereafter, the Captain came on the intercom and said we were going to practice a drill: we were instructed to put on our Mae Wests, to take all pencils and pens out of our pockets, and, at his command, place our heads against the back of the seat in front of us.

This was the first Jo and the children knew of the trouble. It was clear to everyone that this was not a drill at all. We were obviously flying slower and losing altitude. A door in the back of the plane had been opened, and the flight attendants were madly throwing out items from the kitchen in the back of the plane. Fortunately, the bar was situated in the front of the plane.

The Captain again came on the intercom and announced that we would have to land in the ocean. A quick look out the window revealed huge waves. The thought of landing in them was terrifying. The flight attendants directed our attention to the dinghies stored overhead, and informed us very matter-of-factly that once we landed, the dinghies would be inflated and dropped in the water. Our job was to exit the plane, climb out onto the wing and jump down into them. We agreed that Jo would take the two girls out one side, I would take the two boys out the other. We were terribly worried, but did our best to hide our panic from the children. The rest of the passengers on board seemed to be doing the same. There was no hysteria, only the quiet whispers of prayers, and the scribbling sounds of people hurriedly making out their wills.

As we prepared to ditch, the Captain reassured us that

the Coast Guard and all ships in the area had been notified of our unexpected arrival. Those last moments were interminable. I was saying my prayers, when suddenly the Captain again came on the intercom, this time with better news. We were about 300 miles from the island of Hilo and there was a WWII landing strip there; the Captain thought there was a chance we could make it. The next thing we knew we were on a direct approach, flying low and fast. In order to slow us down, the Captain reversed the other engines. One of them caught fire and we descended in a cloud of smoke and flames. However, the fire was quickly put out, the plane rolled to a stop and we slid off in the emergency chutes. No one was hurt but I sure was scared. Billy, who should have been old enough to know better, was delighted with the adventure and couldn't understand why his father was so pale. His comment, "Gee, Dad, you look awfully white!" was quite an understatement.

The Captain later informed us that we'd had less than one minute of fuel remaining. We were transferred to small planes to take us on to Honolulu, and landed in the midst of television cameras and reporters. We left almost immediately for Tokyo, with a brief stop at Midway Island, where we could see remnants of Japanese and U.S. planes in the water and on the ground.

Home at Last

Our arrival in Tokyo was something of an anti-climax. The drive from the airport took us right through the worst of the slum areas, which was a bit of a shock. After we settled into the Imperial Hotel, we went for a walk down the Ginza. It was wall-to-wall people, and the strange sights, sounds and smells were new and somewhat overwhelming, especially for the children.

The next morning we boarded a fast train to Hiroshima. Our first look at Hiroshima did not lift our spirits much. All around we saw the vestiges of the bombing. The debris had all been cleaned up, but the city was still only about 65% rebuilt. Scattered here and there a modern building remained standing, interspersed with newly-constructed houses.

Our house was the size of an American two-car garage. What furniture it did contain was old and fairly battered. There was a lot wrong with it, including a leaking roof and what seemed like more than a fair share of rats. We hired two Japanese girls, Takaka-san and Fugika-san, as housekeepers, and a young man as cook. As was the accepted way under the Occupation, we paid each of them the equivalent of $12.00 a month, plus food. After a few weeks of maneuvering on my part, I was able to get us into somewhat better accommodations, which included a fully functioning roof.

At the time I was there, the ABCC had a staff of more than 500 Americans, Australians and Japanese who hailed from universities all over the world. The primary purpose of the Director of the Adult Medical Program was to study the long-term effects of radiation on human beings. How we would go about doing this was largely at our discretion. In theory, this was to be a collaborative effort with the Japanese, but the hematology division that I directed was never well received by the higher echelons of Japanese science. Part of the reason was that the first Director appointed was a colonel in the army. While Lieut. Colonel Carl F. Tessmer may have been a brilliant pathologist, his Army affiliation had to have been off-putting to the Japanese.

Another contributing factor was that the Japanese considered Hiroshima to be out in the boondocks, peopled with country bumpkins. There was a very strict social consciousness, and imperial universities such as Kyushu, Kyoto and Tokyo felt themselves too upper-crust to have any association with the research going on in Hiroshima. This made considerable difference in our ability to recruit young Japanese physicians and scientists for the program. While not openly hostile, I felt strongly that many of the more distinguished Japanese physicians had little respect for the ABCC. As a result, we never got the stamp of approval from the imperial universities, and had little collaboration with the Japanese doctors. This was unfortunate, because we could have benefitted greatly from each other's knowledge.

The truth is, both medically and geographically, we *were* out in the boondocks. With the exception of the ABCC, there was very little medical research occurring in Hiroshima at the time. Hiroshima Medical School had only started during the war, offering a two-year course to train people to go out in the field and treat the wounded. Conditions at the medical school were rustic at best.

Most of the lectures were given in an old, hanger-like building. There was no heat in these buildings, so on cold winter days make-shift heaters were set up. These "heaters" were really large barrels filled with burning wood, scattered strategically throughout the room. I had to admire the Japanese medical students for bearing up under these harsh conditions. I did my best to teach them, though on the coldest winter days I couldn't help but abbreviate my lectures somewhat.

Radiation Was the Least of Our Troubles

Very quickly after reporting to work at the ABCC, I realized the scope of the problem. Leukemia that occurs as a result of radiation cannot be distinguished from leukemia that occurs naturally, so statistics were the only way to make the distinction. Also, we were looking at radiation from two different sources, with two different types of bombs: Hiroshima was hit with a uranium bomb, Nagasaki with a plutonium one. A complicated survey and sorting process was put in place to account for all the variables. Age, sex, location at the time of the bomb, as well as shielding effect were all taken into account. It was a Herculean task. These were the days before computers, but a good deal was accomplished with mechanical sorters and other devices. Because of the intricacy and number of the variables we had to factor in, statistics became a force unto itself. The Statistics Department was headed by Lowell Woodbury, a mathematician.

We were fortunate in that we had a lot of resources at our disposal. The laboratory facilities were excellent, as were the Japanese lab technicians. Though few spoke English, many of us became close friends by the end of my tenure there. Since we were so isolated, we relied heavily upon one another for companionship. Days were focused on the hard work at hand, but many evenings groups would get together for parties or drinks, and weekends were reserved for tennis or special outings. I recorded one such event in my journal from April 1953: "Took a long, bumpy ride down to see cherry trees at Irakuri. Jo, Tommy and most of ABCC Nijimura gang came along. Lots of people there. Picnic by muddy roadside, many drunks filled with saké, they really get wild on it."

Getting Down to Work

The most important source of radiation was gamma rays. However, people close to ground zero were killed by blast and heat. This accounted for from 70 to 80% of the casualties. About 20% of the victims died of radiation; these were people in cement buildings and otherwise shielded from the initial blast and heat. As one traveled farther out from the hypocenter, the dose of radiation fell off rapidly and averaged about twenty-five rads at the 2000 meter distance. Our job was to study the survivors.

The Japanese did a comprehensive census in 1948, the results of which Grant Taylor was given when he became Director in 1950. We notified everyone on this list to come to the ABCC to be tested. Each participant would receive an increased rice ration. Not surprisingly, about 80% agreed. We set up clinical facilities and planned to see from ten to twenty patients per day. We did chest X-rays, blood studies, chemistries, as well as complete histories for both radiated and non-irradiated patients. I supervised most of these exams, assisted by a number of younger physicians.

Leukemias had to be qualified in order to be accepted

for our study, and accuracy was critical to the study's success. There would be reports of leukemias from Nagasaki, the location of the other half of the ABCC outfit, but no specific diagnoses were made down there. I was anxious to see what was going on, so shortly after settling in Hiroshima I made the trip to Nagasaki. There I met Robert Lange, an accomplished graduate of Washington University in St. Louis, sitting behind a desk, fairly mad with boredom. The operation was not well-organized, and they had few cases to study. It seemed a waste of time to have him down there when I had so much work to do back in Hiroshima. I convinced Dr. Taylor to have Bob join me, knowing that together we could review all the leukemias, both those in Hiroshima and in Nagasaki. Bob was delighted to come, and I was thrilled to have him.

Together we gathered and reanalyzed the data from Nagasaki and wrote the second article ever on radiation-induced leukemia in the survivors. It was published in two parts in the journal *Blood*. Part I described physical characteristics of the Hiroshima bomb, explaining why it acted the way it did. Part II described the clinical and hematological effects of the bomb. The only concrete conclusion we arrived at was the obvious correlation between distance from the bomb and radiation dose. I went on to publish six or seven additional articles on the subject.

Even though the studies were well organized, we still had to deal with certain unknowns and variables. The biggest variable was the radiation doses. Getting an accurate measurement of the levels of radiation received was still ambiguous, and to a certain extent still is today. A shielding study was underway to ascertain the difference in dosage received if the victim was in a flimsy Japanese house, or the same distance away from the epicenter but in a concrete building. Since the study had not yet been completed, and in order to have at least some measurable standards, we used distance as a measure of radiation doses.

This turned out to be as good a method as any; even when completed, the shielding study remained a matter of controversy. It later had to be entirely recalculated when the neutron flux was discovered. It was ironic that our work at the ABCC was in part responsible for the discovery of the neutron flux. We had little knowledge about nuclear physics, yet our findings in Hiroshima and Nagasaki raised questions which had no apparent answer.

Discovering the Neutron Flux

Comparative studies were being done in Hiroshima and Nagasaki since the Hiroshima bomb had been a uranium one and the Nagasaki bomb had been made of plutonium. In Hiroshima, children and young adults were developing cataracts. This was surprising, because you don't expect cataracts in children. In addition, it took a dose of two to three hundred rads before cataracts developed, yet many of these patients had only received twenty-five rads, a very low dose.

David Cogan from the Massachusetts Eye and Ear Infirmary in Boston came out as part of an ophthalmologist group to study these children. We knew the lens of the eye was sensitive to radiation, and especially sensitive to the neutron effect. We also knew that neutrons were more cataractogenic than ordinary x-rays or gamma rays. But that was as much of the puzzle as we could piece together. We asked the physicists what was going on, but they didn't know. Eventually they detonated a small uranium bomb in the desert for study. It was only then, since they knew what to look for, that they were able to measure a neutron flux.

The Genetics Department

In addition to the Hematology Department, there were several other departments under the umbrella of the Atomic Bomb Casualty Commission. The Pathology Department was headed by Bernie Black-Schaffer, a well-known pathologist. The Pediatric Department as well as the Growth and Development Department was staffed by some well-trained young American pediatricians. But the most outstanding and effective department out there was the Genetics Department under the direction of Jack Schull. This group had an unbeatable combination of strong medical ability and management savvy. It was the latter, I'm sure, that was the key to their success.

Schull was an outstanding fellow and with his mentor, Jim Neel, put together a great team of human geneticists. Jim Neel was politically astute, and he arranged through his Washington contacts to develop close relationships with the best geneticists in Japan. From the beginning and throughout the history of the ABCC, this close association operated on a high academic and scientific level, something sadly lacking in other areas of the Casualty Commission's activities.

They were there to study birth defects and genetic defects in irradiated populations. They looked at 86,000

Japanese kids over a period of about five years, and published a monograph which is a classic. It showed that there were no significant genetic defects in the first generation of children born to mothers and fathers who were irradiated. They checked all the permutations: mother irradiated/father not; father irradiated/mother not; as well as those couples who received no radiation. Interestingly, they found no increases in leukemia in children exposed in utero. This was in direct contradiction with studies published in England and other places which said that radiation to mothers caused increases in leukemia and various types of malignancies.

The method they used for managing the study was ingenious. About 95% of babies were delivered by midwives. Midwives had a union, and James and Jack met with the head of the union, and told her that the pregnant women would get an increased rice ration, as well as other perks, if they agreed to participate in the study. So each time a baby was born, one of the midwives would call up to the ABCC. Then one of the geneticists would corral any of the cadre of Japanese doctors and nurses they had standing by for just such an event, and off they would go to make a house call. The baby would be weighed and measured. They'd look for any classical defects, such as too many fingers, an imperforate anus, cleft palate or any visible gross abnormalities. They would also take information from the mother. If the baby died or had been born dead, the midwives put the child in a little shoebox and brought it up to the Commission's laboratories for an autopsy. When the healthy babies were nine months old, they all came back to the clinic for follow-up. Once again the children were measured and studied, this time by the pediatric group.

Trouble at Home

The genetics group made great progress in their research in large part because they were systematic about seeing as many newborns as possible. But what we Americans thought of as organized and efficient, others interpreted as callous and opportunistic. We were getting a lot of negative press in Japan and even in the United States.

Eleanor Roosevelt came to visit, along with some well-known politicians. Even they were influenced by the negative publicity. It was startling to hear Eleanor Roosevelt accuse us of using the survivors as medical guinea pigs. Much as we explained, over and over, that we were there as scientists to assess the biological damage, it always seemed to get misquoted in the press. The widely-read *Life* magazine published an article recounting the horrors of Hiroshima and Nagasaki, and reported that "here and there is resentment against the U.S., but, curiously, it is not because the A bombs were used; rather it is because, as the wife of a much-scarred survivor said, 'If you Americans bombed us, and some of us survived, don't you think . . . you should help us regain our health?' This group claims that the Atomic Bomb Casualty Commission, whose primary task is the study of the long-range effect of atomic bombing, has treated survivors as 'guinea pigs'."

Science magazine took a different slant on our work,

reporting in December of 1952: "It is also a tribute to American sympathy for human suffering that one of the earliest activities of the occupation forces in Japan was the careful study of the survivors of Hiroshima and Nagasaki bombings and the instruction by American physicians of their Japanese colleagues in all the advances in medicine that had been made in this country during the war. Thus, many of the injured survived who would otherwise have died."

Unfortunately, many more Americans read *Life* magazine than read *Science*. As a result, citizens and politicians alike began to think poorly of us. I wrote in my journal January 9, 1953: "They misquote Grant at every turn, and make us look like S.O.B.s no matter what we do." So widespread was this misconception that even those who were supposed to know better believed it. When Eleanor Roosevelt came to Hiroshima for a visit, she arrived at our labs fairly fuming. She'd recently visited with some very angry and vocal Japanese. They were anti-ABCC, and filled her head with their beliefs that we should be offering treatment, rather than just conducting research. We gave Mrs. Roosevelt a tour, and once she saw the set-up, it became clear even to her that we did not have the facilities to treat all 150,000 survivors. It was enough, we felt, to diagnose them and send them back to their own doctors for treatment.

By early 1953, I was beginning to feel we'd hit our stride, and wrote in my journal: "Now that we are getting the data out, it is more exciting. I think we will have a field day with the hematology . . . Also the radiation should be interesting. Breeden is working on the blood pressure problem, Gene will do the tuberculosis, all of us will work on the general diagnoses and sort out the disease groups."

While we were able to make progress on the leukemia, the rest of the diseases we so diligently worked to sort out never crystallized into much. They remained a "soup" of information, none of it coming out as meaning anything. That, combined with ongoing political issues, began to make my time out there frustrating. In July of 1953 I wrote: "I do not see eye to eye with Grant on the research plans. I think he is too cautious and does not demand results. Too many people have been out here without the desire or ability to do clinical research. We have so many differences of opinion that I think it will mean a break in our relationships — it has already altered them."

Grant had the difficult task of appeasing the politicians while at the same time keeping all the research on track. In retrospect, given that the ABCC was actually run by three committees, it may not have been possible at all. In August 1953 entries into my journal again reflected my frustration: "Still trying to get a major attitude adjustment from Committee on work over here. They must do it in a big way or quit. Dr. Burger (epidemological consultant) does not seem to see the clinical side, they are all preoccupied with policy and genetics. There is no down-to-earth thinking on actual facts as we have found them."

Final Results

Science magazine, as well as the more mainstream *Time* published the results of our efforts in Hiroshima. On March 7, 1955 *Time* quoted from the paper I wrote with Robert D.

Lange in *Blood* about leukemia among Japanese atom-bomb survivors.

> Most people near the center of explosion at Hiroshima and Nagasaki died of heat or blast. Some survived these effects, but got heavy doses of gamma rays and neutrons. In Hiroshima, 750 people who had been within 1,000 meters (3,300 feet) recovered from their radiation sickness and remained apparently well for years. Then an unusual number of them showed symptoms of leukemia. So far, fourteen of the 750 have developed the fatal disease. This is more than 600 times the normal incidence of leukemia in Japan.
>
> Survivors farther from the explosion did not get leukemia so frequently, but even among those nearly two miles away the leukemia rate has been far above normal. Dr. Moloney expects other forms of cancer to appear later, and he suspects that the radioactive fall-out of hydrogen bombs will have even greater cancer-producing effect. His guess is that repeated small exposures because of the fall-out will cause more malignancies than the atom bomb's single big dose."

Science explained our results in more detail in its February 11, 1955 issue:

> In a forthcoming technical article on the leukemogenic effects of ionizing radiation on atomic bomb survivors in Hiroshima, William C. Moloney and Marvin Kastenbaum present evidence leading to the following conclusions:
>
> 1. Among the survivors age and sex have no measurable effect on the incidence of leukemia.

2. The incidence of leukemia is higher for those who were closer to the hypocenter than for those farther away at the time of the bombing.

3. The incidence of leukemia is much higher for those with significant radiation complaints than for those with no significant radiation complaints

4. The difference in the incidence of leukemia between the group with and those without significant radiation complaints is not dependent on the distance from the hypocenter. At all distances where cases of leukemia have been found, the incidence of leukemia is higher among the group with significant radiation complaints.

5. It seems apparent from these observations that in man the leukemogenic dose of single total-body ionizing irradiation must be high and is probably in the order of 200 r.

6. Following the Hiroshima atomic bomb explosion, the neutron flux, as evidenced by biologic effects, was apparently much more extensive and heavier than hitherto estimated. Neutron activity may have been an important leukemoginic factor in atomic bomb survivors.

These are just a few short paragraphs to describe months of collaborative effort and research by many dedicated doctors and staff members. While we did not see as much leukemia as I'd expected, we were still able to learn about the disease. Almost by accident we discovered that the pre-leukemic phase could last anywhere from weeks to months before crossing over into full-blown leukemia. And the parameters we set for radiation doses—parameters that we were forced to set for lack of a shielding study—still hold to this day.

Sensie Moloney is Leaving

Except for noting the presence of an increased incidence of leukemia, nothing outstanding had come out of the follow-up studies. I felt I had written and learned as much as possible from what I'd seen out there; it was time for me to go home and figure out what it was I was going to do next. As my departure date neared, I began to count the days.

There was a continuous round of farewell parties. Col. Frank Kelleher hosted one of the two parties that were particularly memorable. Frank was one of my good friends from the British Army Medical Corps. These young medical officers, mostly English, Canadian, Australian and New Zealanders, had been drafted to serve for two years during the Korean War. The British Armed Forces were training chiefly in Southern Japan, and had a large military hospital in Kure, the former naval base, about ten miles above Hiroshima. Frank threw a party worthy of all the nationalities who attended: there was saki, geisha girls and party games and dancing. Toward the end of the party I was presented with a beautiful plaque that had been carved out of wood from the Tori, a huge, H-shaped monument set in the inlets of the Inland Sea. When the structure was replaced, the wood was preserved for special objects, and was considered sacred. My plaque stated: "Presented to Dr. W. Moloney by the British Army Medical Corps in recognition of his efforts in conducting rounds and teaching at the ABCC in Hiroshima."

Dr. Hachiya was the host of the other memorable party. Dr. Hachiya was a surgeon and the author of *Hiroshima*, which published the first eyewitness accounts of Hiroshima survivors. The hospital he owned on the outskirts of Hiroshima City was destroyed by the bomb. He himself received a considerable dose of radiation, along with injuries and severe burns. Nevertheless, he earnestly desired friendship between Japan and the United States. Our friendship was genuine, and as his wife danced a traditional tea dance and his son entertained us with a magic show. I knew I would miss him. He presented me with an unusual Japanese plate to commemorate our friendship, saying that he hoped it would remind me of the smiling face of Japan.

Finally, there were no more parties to attend, and my long-anticipated departure date arrived. As I drove down the hill from Nijimora, the road was lined with friends and colleagues bowing and waving goodbye. "Sensie Moloney (professor) is leaving." It was very touching. This moment stood in sharp contrast with my experience aboard the S.S. President Cleveland, the cruise ship I boarded in Tokyo to take me home. The ship was filled with wealthy tourists, most of them on around-the-world cruises. The glitz and glitter, their loud and boisterous antics, I found quite unsettling after spending two years among people who had so few material posessions.

Recall

I pretty much kept to myself, and passed the time reading. I was up on deck when someone came up to tell me I had a cablegram. It was the head of the Atomic Energy Commission cabling me to turn around and return to Hiroshima as quickly as I could. The H-bomb "Bravo" had been detonated over Bikini Atoll in the Marshall Islands. Winds had shifted and fallout was raining down on the natives and servicemen peopling the Marshall Islands. An unlucky group of fisherman, aboard the inappropriately named "Fuku Moru" (Lucky Dragon) had drifted into the detonation area and received high doses of radiation (200–300 rads). Because of the natives' habit of covering their bodies with sticky coconut oil, the fallout clung to their skin. The exposure caused anemia, thrombocytopenia and leukopenia, which Japanese doctors treated incorrectly with small repeated blood transfusions. One sailor developed severe serum hepatitis which resulted in fatal liver damage.

His death was inaccurately attributed to radiation. The newspapers picked up the story and people panicked. Dr. Shields Warren, a noted pathologist, obtained slides from this sailor's autopsy which gave clear evidence that the death was caused by serum hepatitis. Nevertheless, the *Bulletin of Atomic Scientists* and the noted *Manchester Guardian* ran lurid accounts of the death and attributed it to radiation.

I was infuriated by the flagrant mistruths printed. The feeling would not be short-lived. This was the first of many recurring instances of the media scaring the public. By the time nuclear energy plants began proliferating, there was a deep-seated, though unwarranted, fear of radiation. On every occasion, even a small bit of waste from a nuclear plant was exaggerated to a frightening degree. A prime example was the alarmist publicity surrounding the Three Mile Island incident. This event could have been catastrophic, no doubt about that. But, because of the good design of this reactor (the error leading to the melt-down was a human one), the fire in the nuclear fuel was contained and eventually smothered. Practically no nuclear emission occurred outside the plant. No one was injured or killed in the accident.

Chernobyl

Similar exaggeration occurred over the Chernobyl accident. This was no doubt a major disaster, caused by a combination of human error and a poorly designed nuclear reactor. 237 individuals had immediate radiation effects, and 134 suffered from radiation sickness. Of the 134 acute cases, twenty-eight died (two of injuries at the site). In a report published in *Spectrum* in November 1996, ten deaths occurred in survivors over the past ten years, though these deaths were not necessarily due to radiation. In this article and several other reports on childhood leukemia published in Europe, it is noted that over the past ten years there has been no detectable increase in the incidence of leukemia or cancer. Yet little of this information is reported in the popular press.

Shortly after the Chernobyl accident, an emergency meeting was convened at the Brookhaven National Laboratory under the supervision of Dr. Eugene Cronkite. A large number of experts on the effects of ionizing radiation attended, mostly from the United States as well as a number from Europe, especially Germany. But the Russians refused to have the U.S. participate in their clean-up efforts. They would only allow Armand Hammer to send Robert Peter Gale over with medical supplies. Dr. Gale attempted, with Russian colleagues, to do bone marrow transplants on ten heavily irradiated workers. It was a pathetic effort. The

facilities at the Moscow hospital were primitive, so they
were unable to type white blood cells for complete matches,
and they took anybody with ABO compatibility. Within
twenty-four to forty-eight hours the classic radiation symptoms began: nausea, vomiting and bleeding from the gums,
with things going downhill from there. All ten of these
workers died, though amazingly, others received almost as
much exposure, 200–300 rads, and survived.

I learned a possible explanation some years later when,
in 1970, I was asked to consult on an Etiology of Cancer
project sponsored by the International Agency for Research. We studied 90,000 patients with cervical cancer who
had been treated with radium and X-ray to the lower
abdomen. I reviewed all the leukemia cases. Our surprising
finding was that the increased risk of developing leukemia
from radiation was relatively low. The estimated risk at
1 Gy (100 rads) was 1.7. This low risk was attributed by
Boice to cell killing, and Cronkite and Bond pointed out
that bone marrow stem cells migrated in and out of the
marrow. Both these discoveries were possible explanations
for the low incidence of leukemia in these patients.

We now know that ionizing radiation, from a variety of
sources, can cause leukemia. However, there is no experimental or epidemiological evidence that doses below 25
rads produce the disease. The overall numbers of chronic
myelocytic leukemia and acute leukemia caused by radiation are small and probably represent less than 1% of all
human leukemias.

A Japanese paper recently published in the *National
Cancer Review* claims radiation is a strong leukemogen, with
effects remaining from forty to fifty years after exposure.

In truth, radiation is not a strong leukemogen, and there is no evidence of such long-term effect. For the most part, radiation-induced leukemias appear from ten to fifteen years following exposure. Very little information has come out of Russia on studies of the Chernobyl survivors. Of course, there have been the usual "the sky is falling" reports about fallout. But except for an increase in thyroid tumors, as was the case in the Marshall Islands, thus far we have not seen any late radiation effects from Chernobyl.

Recall Rebuff

I decided to ignore the AEC cablegram directing me back to Japan to study the fallout on the Fuku Mora crew. Granted, the work could have been interesting, but I was fed up with being managed by a committee of committees thousands of miles away. I made up my mind that I was not going back. As things would turn out, later in my career I would spend some time in the Marshalls studying the effects of this fallout. But for now, my contract had been completed and I was going home. When I got to San Francisco, I took the longest route home that I could. I knew if I went directly back to Boston "they" would find me. So I took the scenic route, stopping in Texas to interview Neil Wald as my possible replacement.

A fitting end to my trip was the journey from San Antonio to Houston, during which we encountered a problem. I couldn't believe it when the pilot made the announcement to prepare for an emergency landing. It seems I'd heard those very words at the beginning of the trip. The only saving grace was that now I felt myself a veteran, and knew what to do. Fortunately, this landing was not very dramatic. The pilot had noticed fuel leaking, and it turned out that someone had replaced the gas cap incorrectly. The trip continued without further incident. And, as I had suspected (and hoped), by the time I got home others had been sent out to study the unfortunate fisherman.

As far as my career was concerned my stint in Japan provided the breakthrough I had hoped for. Even though the anticipated hoards of leukemia cases never materialized, I did not feel my work in Japan was for naught. Some of our studies on chronic myelogeous leukemia, especially the absence of leukocyte alkaline phosphatase in polymorphonuclear leukocytes of patients with early phases of the disease, did provide insight into certain characteristics of chronic myelogeous leukemia granulocytes. Once I returned to Boston I was considered an expert on radiation effects. I was put on some rather prestigious committees, and all kinds of groups asked me to participate in their leukemia studies.

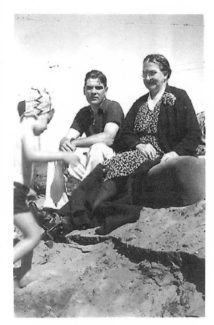

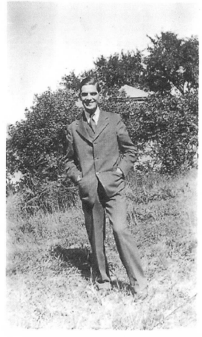

Illustration 1 (above): William C. Moloney (center) with mother (right) and daughter Patsy (left), Nantucket, 1938. Illustration 2 (below): WCM photographed during his senior year at Tufts Medical School, 1932.

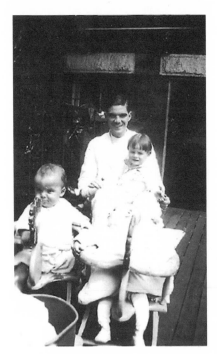

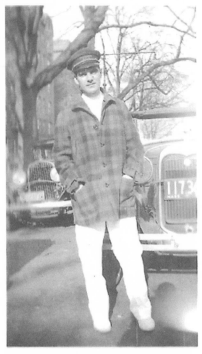

Illustration 3 (above): WCM in 1931, with children he delivered at St. Mary's Infant Asylum, while a medical student. Illustration 4 (below): WCM on ambulance duty at Kings County Hospital, Brooklyn, N.Y., 1932.

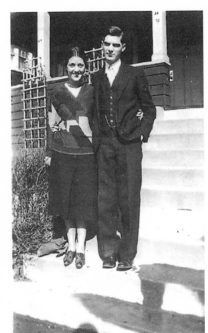

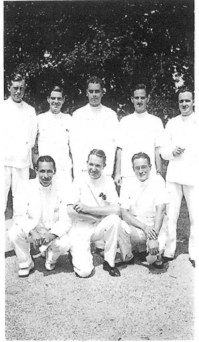

Illustration 5 (above): WCM with wife Josephine, 1932. The couple met at a party during WCM's second year of medical school and had secretly married. Illustration 6 (below): The Kings County House Officers, 1932. WCM is in the second row, second from left.

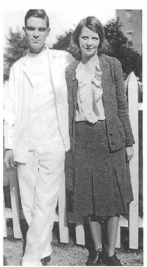

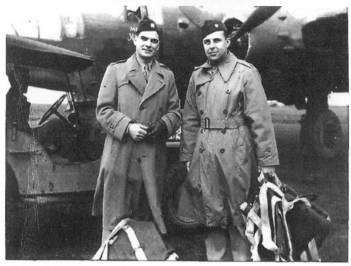

Illustration 7 (above): WCM with a 23-year-old patient with Friedreich's ataxia, who died shortly after the picture was taken. Illustration 8 (below): WCM (left) in England, 1944, prior to the invasion of Europe. After a flight in bad weather, during which he was ordered to prepare to jump—(the pilot was able to land the plane safely)—"I found myself making a vow I would repeat throughout my life: 'I am never again getting on an airplane'."

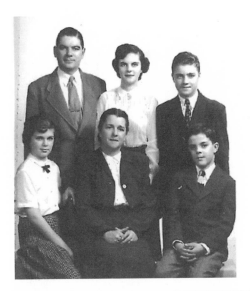

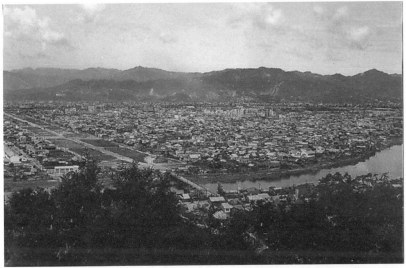

Illustration 9 (above): The Moloney family posed for a passport picture prior to their trip to Japan, 1952. Front row, left to right, Elizabeth, Josephine, and Billy; back row, WCM, Patsy and Tommy. Illustration 10 (below): Hiroshima, pictured at the time when the Moloney's first arrived in Japan. The view is from the Atomic Bomb Casualty Commission's clinic, on the hill above the city.

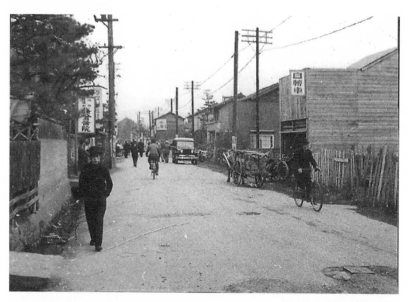

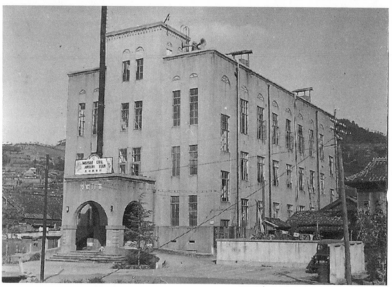

Illustration 11 (above): A typical street in Nagasaki. Illustration 12 (below): Atomic Bomb Casualty Commissions laboratory in Nagasaki.

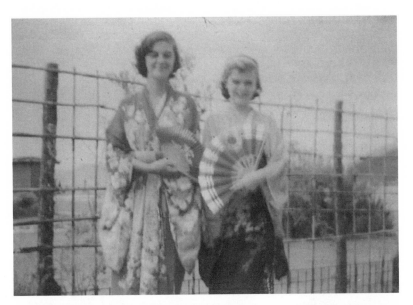

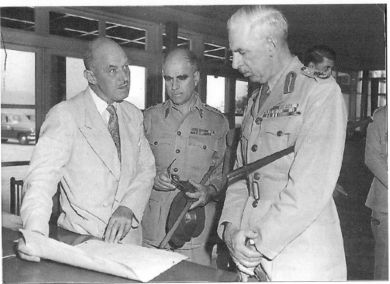

Illustration 13 (above): Patsy and Elizabeth in Japanese costume, 1952. Illustration 14 (below): British Medical College VIPs "checking us out".

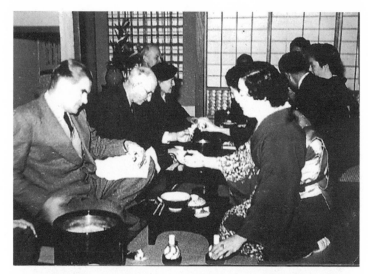

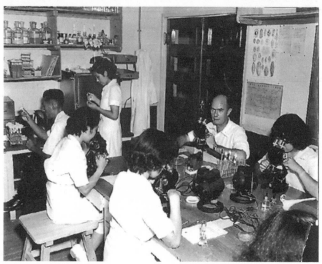

Illustration 15 (above): Japanese party in honor of John Morin, Professor of Surgery at Rochester, who replaced Grant Taylor as Director of the Atomic Bomb Causalty Commission. Illustration 16 (below): Tax Cornell, from Dartmouth Medical School, headed the parasitology laboratory of the Atomic Bomb Casualty Commission.

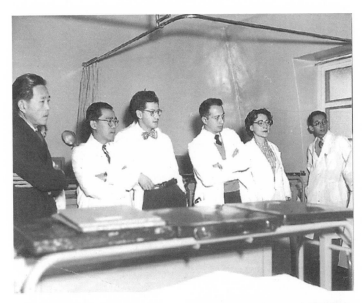

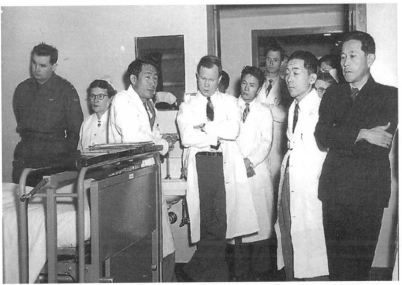

Illustration 17 (above): Rounds at the Atomic Bomb Casualty Commission, Hiroshima. Illustration 18 (below): Rounds with the Royal Army Medical Corps.

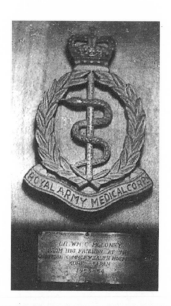

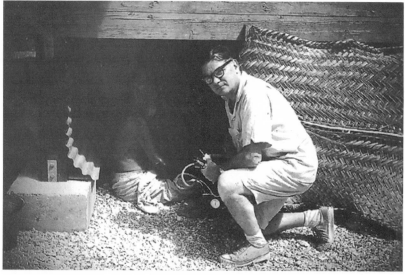

Illustration 19 (above): Teaching award presented to WCM by the Royal Army Medical Corps. Illustration 20 (below): WCM making an "under the house call" in the Marshall Islands, 1962.

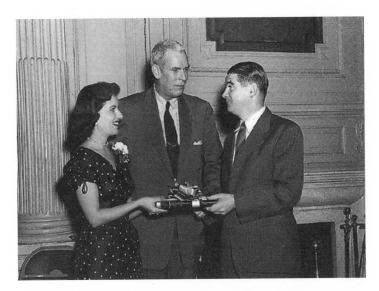

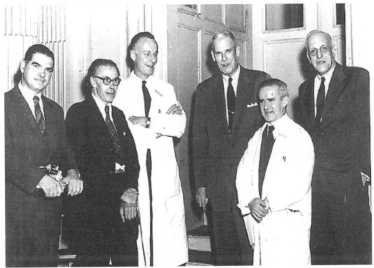

WCM becomes Director of Laboratories at Boston City Hospital, July 1954. Illustration 21 (above): "They gave me the present *before* Superintendent Conlon told me that I would be in charge of the labs." Illustration 22 (below): WCM with staff of the Harvard Unit at Boston City Hospital. Left to right, WCM, F. H. Laskey Taylor, Charles S. Davidson, John Conlon, Maxwell Finland, William B. Castle.

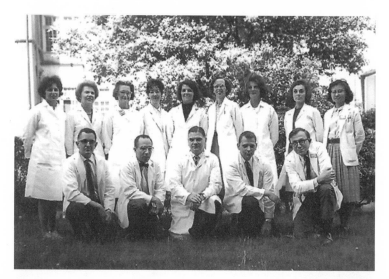

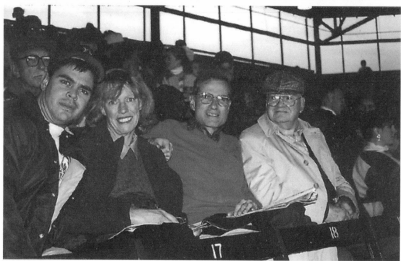

Illustration 23 (above): The staff of the Tufts Hematology Lab, 1964–1965. WCM is in the center of the front row, and James Desforges is behind him in the second row, sixth from the left. Illustration 24 (below). At Fenway Park for a Red Sox game, 1995. WCM (far right), Frank Bunn (beside him), Betsy Bunn, and the Bunns' son George.

Chapter Six

RATS, HAWKS and DOVES

1954–1966

AT FOUR O'CLOCK in the morning I stood in the Operating Room holding tight to the hand of a 14 year-old boy as he lay on the operating table, struggling for breath. It was intensely frustrating to me that simple compassion was the only weapon left in my arsenal against Hodgkins disease.

The only son of a widowed mother, John Garabedian had Hodgkins disease. We treated him with local x-ray, one of the few therapies available to us at the time, and the lymph nodes receded. But only temporarily. The nodes re-enlarged, and other classic Hodgkins symptoms began: soaking night sweats, fever and weight loss. A course of Nitrogen Mustard (NH_2) was effective, then John began to have difficulty breathing. X-ray showed the lymph nodes in his chest had enlarged to the point that they were compressing the bronchial tubes. We realized that excision was probably hopeless, but the thoracic surgeons thought it worth a try. In truth, it was his only chance.

Opening John's chest revealed a huge mass of white fibrous tissue. His wind pipe was fully surrounded, making it impossible for the surgeon to open an airway. John took a few last strangled breaths then died. His mother was devastated, but understood we'd done everything possible. For several years after his death she worked an extra job selling nylon stockings just so she could contribute money for our research work. With her small sums we purchased special medical texts and placed a marker in each book in John's honor. I recently ran across some of these books in our Hematology Library at the Brigham and Women's Hospital. Seeing the dedication brought back sad memories. Most tragic is that just a few years later we would have had an 80% chance of putting John into remission.

Boston City Hospital and the Tufts Hematology Lab

Following my stint as Director of the Atomic Bomb Casualty Commission, I was offered the position of Chief of Laboratories at Boston City Hospital. Attendant with this position was a promotion to Clinical Professor of Medicine, as well as Chief of the 3rd Medical Service (Tufts), and Physician to the Boston City Hospital. The salary was $15,000 per year, and the laboratories I would oversee included the Blood Bank and the Biochemical Lab, as well as the smaller service laboratories. I was grateful to have F.H. Laskey Taylor appointed head of the Biochemical Laboratory, since this was not my field of expertise.

Dr. Biguria and Jane Desforges were delighted to have me back. Jane had acted as the chief during my absence. "Biggy" couldn't wait to show me what was to be our new research facility, and proudly led me over to the old Sears Surgical Pavilion. It was a grand old place. Or at least it once had been. Ceilings soared twenty feet, floors were marble, and intricate woodwork predominated. It was something out of Victorian England, and just about as old. Dust covered everything, plaster fell from the ceiling at fairly regular intervals, and paint was peeling from the grime-covered walls. In spite of this, it represented some much-needed space. We organized an extensive clean up, then set about improvising laboratory benches and fitting out the smaller rooms as offices and examining rooms. Though a bit ramshackle, the Tufts Hematology Laboratory was open for business.

A year or so after our "new" labs were up and running, I was not at all surprised to enter the room one morning to see John Kenney, one of my fellows, sitting at his desk holding an open umbrella, seemingly unperturbed by the stream of water pouring down from the leaky roof. Such was life at BCH.

Isotopes at ORINS

My job as Chief of Labs included overseeing the isotope lab. This obliged me to learn a thing a two about isotopes. At that time, radioactive gold and other isotopes were injected into patients as treatment for various forms of metastatic cancer. They were beginning to have some success, and everyone seemed to feel this would be the way to go to cure cancer. The Oak Ridge Institute for Nuclear Studies (ORINS) in Tennessee had a small, twelve-bed facility to which patients were referred for the use of these experimental protocols. I'd only been home from Japan a few weeks when I left for a three-month course at ORINS to obtain practical experience in the use of diagnostic and therapeutic radioisotopes. Though the course work was difficult, I spent an enjoyable three months there and was able to earn my license to handle radioactive material.

This license made me an instant expert. As such, once back in Boston I was put in charge of making sure that all of the radioactive material throughout Boston City Hospital was stored properly. The inspections I performed were by no means gratuitous. One day the Geiger counter almost jumped out of my hand. I walked into the room to find a radioactive source sitting on a bench, completely unshielded. Another time, I passed a woman sitting in the waiting room, minding her own business, when the needle on the counter again went off the scale. I gave the woman a second look, and, as surreptitiously as I could, knelt down to have a look beneath her. It turned out that space was short in the storage facility so the patient waiting room was pinch-hitting as the radioactive isotopes storage area. After that, everybody got much better about storing things properly.

Once I was denied entry to the Thorndike for inspection. I told the rather haughty doctor barring my way that it was his choice: either I could do the inspection or someone from the government would be called in to do it. He held his ground, and said coolly: "Only Thorndike members are allowed into the lab." This was ridiculous, and it only took one call to William Castle put things right again. But it really showed me how territorial people could be about their research. This was especially frustrating at a time when what was needed was more dissemination of research results, not less.

Always on Call

If someone had held a Geiger counter up to me in those days, the needle probably would have jumped off the scale. This was a busy time for me. I was running the labs and maintaining my practice at Bay State Road while trying to fulfill the increasing number of consultation requests which came in from every hospital within a thirty-mile radius of Boston. The majority of the cases I saw were diagnostic problems: cases of aplastic anemia, ideopathic thrombocytopenia purpura (ITP), infectious monunucleosis, various types of bleeding disorders and hemolytic anemia. A small percentage of the cases I saw were malignancies: acute and chronic leukemia, malignant lymphoma (lymphosarcoma), multiple myeloma and Hodgkins disease. My chief interests were the cases of acute and chronic leukemia, the malignant lymphatic disorders, Hodgkin's disease, and multiple myeloma.

Off I would go, at all hours, always with my trusty bone marrow needle, an early version of the bone marrow aspirator needle, secure in my front pocket. My ability to obtain and interpret bone marrow specimens was one of my chief claims to fame. As it became known that I was one of the few doctors with this skill, my reputation grew. The result? More consultation requests. We still had just one car, and I put more miles on that old blue Dodge than the manufacturer ever intended.

Bone marrow aspiration only became widely practiced in the late 1930s; I first learned about it while a student at Tufts, enrolled in William Dameshek's hematology class. At that time, almost all bone marrow specimens were obtained from the sternum or breast bone. However, the sternum is a relatively thin bone, 1/2 to 3/4 inches thick, and a needle could easily penetrate through the sternum into the mediastinum and occasionally into the pleural cavity. More rarely, a marrow needle punctured the heart itself with fatal results.

Many diseases would not lend themselves to aspiration, either because it wasn't possible to get to the cells, or because there were not any cells to extract. So I'd do a bone marrow biopsy by incising down to bone and removing a button of bone and marrow. The marrow particles were smeared on glass slides and the rest of the specimen placed in a fixative solution. The fixed specimens were then cut and stained for microscopic examination. It was surprising to find in many instances an "empty" peripheral blood but a marrow filled with malignant cells. This was just one of many mysteries.

Some Progress

Any type of hematological malignancy was, with few exceptions, fatal. At that time Hodgkins disease was especially distressing. It was rare in children and old people, but common in teenagers and young adults. The disease typically progressed quickly and terminated in a miserable fashion. To see otherwise healthy, young individuals die in this manner was horrendous for all involved. Local treatment with the available low-voltage X-ray machine did cause shrinkage of large lymphatic masses close to the surface of the skin, but the machines were not yet powerful enough to get radiation below the surface of the skin. Trying to treat masses in the chest and abdomen with increased voltage only resulted in a bad skin burn. Nitrogen Mustard (NH_2), which had been found to give temporary remissions, was the only other treatment we had to offer.

The usefulness of Nitrogen Mustard was discovered by serendipity. It was developed for use in World War I, but employed by neither the Germans nor ourselves. However, supplies of NH_2 were carried to Europe and in 1944 a ship carrying a supply of it sunk in an Italian harbor. Members of the crew were thrown into the water and, once in the hospital, astute observers called attention to their lowered white counts, lowered platelet counts and anemia. Pharmacologists carried out lab studies which confirmed that NH_2 was capable of suppressing blood forming elements in the bone marrow. This was a significant finding.

Trials were organized in several centers around the country and it was soon discovered that NH_2 had a remarkable effect on Hodgkin's disease. Treatment results were dramatic. The fever would come down with a bang, the nodes would shrink and you'd think the patient cured. But the remissions were relatively brief, lasting anywhere from weeks to months, and the disease resisted further therapy. The question then became how to prolong the remission. It was difficult to treat leukemia and allied diseases because little was known about the biology of malignant bone marrow cells. The cause of malignant cell transformation was not known, nor was there knowledge of the regulations of cell growth and maturation. A series of discoveries yielded insight, but not answers. George Minot had earlier carried out studies on chronic myelogeous leukemia and had been able to achieve remission by irradiating the enlarged spleen and the bone marrow. However, remissions were short and when the disease relapsed, it occurred usually in a very acute form known as "blast cell crisis." This phase of the disease did not respond to therapy; death always followed quickly. Earlier attempts at chemotherapy had employed an arsenical in the form of Fowlers solution. However, the dose required to control the white count was at a toxic level. Other compounds such as urethane were also tried but proved ineffective.

In 1951, Fred Stohlmann and others discovered that red cell proliferation was controlled by the growth factor erythropoietin. This was the first step in understanding how primitive cells matured. This same year Alexander Haddow in London produced a drug known as Myleran (busulfan). This was an alkylating agent and could be administered by mouth. Myleran was very effective in bringing down elevated white counts and shrinking enlarged spleens. It produced remissions in a large percentage of cases of CML but these patients always relapsed and developed a terminal blast cell crisis. Moreover, Myleran had some nasty side effects, cataracts and pulmonary fibrosis among them.

Other investigators in the United States, England, Australia and Germany began studies on cell proliferation. Soon, information was forthcoming on cell cycling and cellular differentiation. These discoveries led to development of new chemotherapeutic agents that could block cell proliferation. One of the earlier agents was 6-mercaptopurine, an inhibitor of purine metabolism. This agent could be administered orally, and produced remission in some patients. However, only a small percentage of patients responded, and for those who did, the remissions were short.

I thought clues could be found in the enzymes in white cells. An article by Valentine and Beck intrigued me, and I spent a day with them learning how to separate out white cells and measure the amount of alkaline phosphatase. At Oak Ridge I learned how to do this test histochemically, and for a brief while this was yet another test I was called upon to administer. This test was short-lived, however. The discovery of chromosomes proved to be a better indicator.

Some Dogs, Many Rats

During the early 1950s I focused my research on these enzymes. Working with Eve Wiltshire and John Kenney, my research fellows at BCH, we conducted numerous experiments to find out anything more we could about cell proliferation. We soon realized that our efforts to study leukemia in man were too limited to be useful, so we turned to animal research. Even though we had only a few animal cages at the BCH, we began studies on leukemia in the rat. We opted to use white rats, rather than mice, because, during my work at Oak Ridge I had noted that the blood producing cells in the rat bone marrow were very similar to the human, much more so than the dog or mice. This got me looking into the estereses and other enzymes in leukemic white cells. I was searching for any kind of clue as to what made the leukemic white cell different from a healthy white cell. To the eye, they looked the same.

This research did yield some important information, specifically, the differences between normal myeloid and leukemic myeloid cells. Leukocyte alkaline phosphatase, identified by histochemical methods, proved to be of some value in distinguishing normal from leukemic polymorphonuclear leukocytes. But while we were getting some interesting information in the lab, our patients continued to die. The research provided no improvement to our patient care, nor yielded any new insight into the basic causes of leukemia.

Nevertheless, our research caught the attention of J. Engelbert Dunphy, Professor of Surgery at Harvard Medical School and Chief of the Fifth Surgical Service at BCH. Bert was an old friend from before the war, when we had worked together at the Holy Ghost. He was in every respect an outstanding scholar, surgeon, and humanitarian. One of Bert's many research projects was transplanting dog kidneys to a subcutaneous location in the neck. Preliminary efforts were not successful, and it was suggested he precede the kidney transplant with a bone marrow transplant. Stanley Jacob, one of Bert's younger fellows, wandered over to our little lab to talk to me about the feasibility of this. I was not optimistic. At that time, little was known about transplants of bone and marrow to other sites within the same individual. I was not optimistic about the results, but I promised Bert I'd contribute what I could.

Dunphy and I set about figuring out how to get bone marrow to proliferate in areas that would be accessible for harvesting. We removed sections of dog rib, sharpened the ends and inserted the ribs into a variety of test sites: the subcutaneous tissue, muscle, liver, spleen and kidney. We followed the transplants with biopsies along with smears of the material, and found that bone and marrow together grew well in the spleen, kidney and psoas muscle, but rib sections transplanted to the liver and subcutaneous sites failed to grow. Since the spleen in the dog had a long pedicle, we used that as our primary site for growing bone and marrow.

Once the transplant took, we gave the dog a lethal dose of NH_2. But just prior to administering it, we clamped off the splenic pedicle with a soft clamp. The clamp was released immediately after the NH_2 was administered and, much to our gratification, the bone marrow continued to grow well in the spleen while the bone marrow that had come in contact with the NH_2 was wiped out. The protected marrow from the spleen continued to grow. As we followed these animals we noted that the general marrow cavity became completely repopulated from the surviving marrow in the spleen. This research gave me a solid understanding of the changes in cell biology when transferred from one site to another. Stanley Jacob, Bert Dunphy and I published several papers on the topic.

Unfortunately, Dunphy's program ended just as quickly as it began. Bert left Harvard to take the position of Chief of Surgery at the University of California in San Francisco. But I was not willing to give up on what I thought were promising experiments. I decided to conduct an identical

study on white rats. Since we could no longer avail ourselves of the plush animal facility run by the Harvard
Services at BCH, I set up a research program in a lab at
the Holy Ghost Hospital.

The first part of this research entailed establishing two
groups of rats, one group with spleens, the other group
with spleens removed. A noted chest surgeon agreed to take
out the rats' spleens for us. This is not a technically difficult
procedure, nevertheless all the rats died. We couldn't believe it. It turned out the rats were more difficult to work
with than the dogs. Rats frightened easily, and if mishan-
dled, could die. Or, in our case, did die. More critical than
surgical skills, it seemed, was skill in handling the animals.
We were fortunate to find that skill in Vin King, a first
cousin of my former fellow, Bill Harrington. Vin had been
a hospital corps man in the Navy during World War II. He
had always wanted to go into medicine but was financially
unable to do so. He was doing very well as a cabinetmaker,
but was still determined to get into some medical field. So
at Bill's suggestion, Vin came to see if I could help him
get admitted to medical school.

The year was 1957, and admission to medical school by
that time was difficult. Moreover, Vin had no college cred-
its. I explained to him the impossibility of getting into
medical school, but asked if he'd consider working with me
on the rat study. I took him over to my lab at the Holy
Ghost Hospital and introduced him to my friend, Dr. Shu
Chu Shen. Dr. Shen had a small animal facility where he
was studying the effects of Vitamin B12 and folic acid on
proliferation of red cells in the rat bone marrow. Dr. Shen

showed Vin the fundamentals of rat care, and he rapidly became proficient in handling rats. He quickly learned that if you were gentle with these animals, a lot could be accomplished. The Sisters gave me permission to expand our primitive animal laboratory and Vin, master carpenter and now promising rat surgeon, built cages and laboratory benches. We used to joke that we had more visiting rats than caged ones.

A breakthrough came in my research when I read about Dr. Harry Shay's work at the Wistar Institute in Philadelphia. Dr. Shay had been trying to produce cancer of the stomach in rats, but instead of cancer the rats developed chloromas, green tumors made up of myeloblasts. Dr. Shay produced these chloromas by prolonged feeding, via stomach tube, of a carcinogenic compound known as methylcholanthrene (MCA). After some weeks, his infant rats developed large subcutaneous tumors. When these were removed and sectioned, they appeared green in color, though the color rapidly faded when exposed to air. The cells making up the tumors were very young myeloid cells, i.e. promyelocytes and myeloblasts, the same sort of cells present in human acute myelogenous leukemia. This was exciting. If we could duplicate his results, we would be able to study how the rats got the tumors, and how the cells changed as the tumors developed. This was exactly the information we needed for our leukemia research.

At our request, Dr. Shay kindly sent us two of his chloroma-bearing rats. Using a hollow needle, we took fresh pieces of tumor from Dr. Shay's rats and implanted them subcutaneously to a number of our very young rats.

Much to our delight, these transplants took and several of the recipient rats developed marked swelling of the abdomen. On removing the abdominal fluid we found it to be filled with leukemic promyelocytes and myeloblasts. We continued to transplant these tumors for many years and eventually found that the cells could be preserved by deep freezing. On warming, the cells were found to be viable, and when injected into newborn rats, chloro-leukemia developed.

The Boloney Virus

Based on this research I was invited to participate in a conference at the University of Chicago on the etiology of cancer. My topic was radiation-induced leukemia. I arrived in Chicago in the middle of a raging snowstorm. The wind howled and snow swirled about my face. I pulled my collar up, pushed my hat down and trudged off in search of a cab. I was becoming desperate of ever finding one when, as if in a vision, a chauffeur ran up and asked if I was Dr. Moloney. When I said "yes," he led me to a large limousine. I couldn't have been more pleased. Just as we were about to leave a snow-covered man came running up and asked if he could have a ride into town. I was feeling fairly magnanimous at this point, so said "Sure. Hop in." Once we were on our way he introduced himself as Dr. Moloney. I burst out laughing. Of course. This was the famous John Moloney, who had world-wide recognition for his discovery of the mouse leukemia viruses. They had sent the car for him! Fortunately, John was a very agreeable fellow and didn't kick me out of the car.

After the conference I sent John some of my chloro-leukemic rats. He and his associates found lots of viruses in them, but none that caused leukemia. At John's suggestion I tried growing leukemic cells in cultures, then put the cultures through a cell-free filter. Sure enough, two weeks later all the infant rat recipients developed leukemia. I was elated. Finally, a virus to call my own. Except, what *would* I call it. John Moloney already had three "Moloney viruses." How to distinguish mine? I called John with the good news of my discovery, and posed the problem of what to name it. John gave it careful consideration and came back with, "How about the Boloney Virus?"

It turns out the name was appropriate. Upon double-checking the virus, I saw that the chloro-leukemia was identical in every respect to the original disease. The karyotypes on these cells showed the same marker chromosomes. I sensed something was fishy. We repeated the experiments and found that the filters were permeable to cells. The leukemia hadn't been transferred by virus at all. Disappointed, we carried on, and over the next few years carried out numerous experiments on the rat chloroma and published a number of papers. As a result of these publications we became better known, and attracted the interest of Dr. Sidney Farber, a powerful, well-connected man in charge of the Jimmy Fund, a pediatric unit of Children's Hospital dedicated to malignancies in children. For his latest research, Dr. Farber needed cells from adults with leukemia, and he found out about our work through his assistant, Tom Hall.

I'd known about Dr. Farber since 1946, when he observed that children with acute leukemia treated experimentally with folic acid experienced an acceleration of the disease. Dr. Farber induced Dr. Subbarow in the Harvard Medical School Department of Pharmacology to synthesize false copies of folic acid known as amethopterin. These compounds proved to be, on a temporary basis, remarkably effective in childhood leukemia, though without long-lasting results.

Getting By at Boston City Hospital

With the help and advice from Dr. Farber, I applied for and received an institutional grant of $250,000, which enabled us to move into a relatively new building at the Holy Ghost Hospital and construct a modern animal facility , along with an excellent laboratory, offices and conference rooms. There was also enough money remaining to employ a pathologist, a research fellow and two or three pre-med students as summer interns. We were fortunate to get Anthony Boschetti as our pathologist. He had just finished training at the Mallory Institute and did great work.

Bear in mind that this research, as well as my private practice, was a sideline to my real job of running the Hematology Division at BCH. Boston City Hospital was a wonderful place to work, with a high level of energy, excitement and commitment to teaching. But disappointing was the lack of professional recognition and support from Tufts. Since Tufts admittedly was a school short on finances, they gave us no money for fellows, did not support our research financially or intellectually, and made no attempts to mentor us and promote deserving young physicians to membership in the important clinical research societies.

The field of hematology was rapidly expanding in the 1950s, and societies like the International Society for Hematology and The American Society of Hematology sprang up. These societies were less exclusive than the American Society for Clinical Investigation, and we flooded them with members. These vigorous, democratic and progressive groups provided an excellent forum for our budding young medical research people. The appearance of the journal *Blood*, founded by Bill Dameshek, was also a landmark development that helped make hematology research and advances in technique available to all.

Because we got no support from Tufts, and resources at BCH were slim at best, we utilized interns and residents as our research staff. It was the first time interns and residents were allowed to participate in the research studies that would affect the very patients they were seeing. I was amused to learn later that this approach was seen as revolutionary. At the time, I saw this more as a necessity; it had the benefit of creating a cadre of especially well-trained hematologists who understood the connection between bench and bedside.

Because the interns and residents were given so much responsibility, I made sure they were well-trained. Thus was born the William Moloney Bone Marrow Course. I made up a kit with slides of all the different blood diseases. Once a week I'd give the staff a series of slides to look at, then return in an hour to discuss it with them. This proved to be an effective learning tool, and soon I had a waiting list for the eight-session course. All the hematology fellows and medical residents rotating through the Hematology Division at BCH took the bone marrow course.

More Progress

Leukemia research was carried on around the world and finally, in the late 50s and early 60s, we began to get a sense of real progress. In 1959, Norwell and Hungerford at the University of Pennsylvania discovered that patients with chronic myelogeous leukemia posessed a small (minute) chromosome in the leukemic myeloblasts. This they named the Ph chromosome, and further studies revealed that this minute chromosome was formed by a reciprocal translocation between the long arms of chromosomes 9 and 22; it was consistently present in over 98% of cases of CML. The discovery of this unique marker chromosome led to additional studies which showed that the rearranged portions of the chromosome contained a locus which controlled an important growth-regulating enzyme: tyrosine kinase. Continuing studies of this enzyme may provide additional insights into the growth and regulation of leukemic cells.

Advances were made in the treatment of childhood leukemia with the discovery of prednisone and the antifolic acid compounds. But the management of acute leukemia in adults continues to be particularly frustrating. Leukemia in childhood responds in 80% of cases to these compounds, but we are unable to duplicate these results in adults and young adults. The reason for the difference in response is that 80% of children have lymphoblastic leukemia while 80% of adults have non-lymphatic leukemia. This failure of response to single-agent therapy is particularly unfortunate since the majority of acute myelogeous leukemia (AML) cases occur in young adults.

A small percentage of adults with acute lymphatic leukemia (ALL) may obtain remission with prednisone and the anti-folic acid compounds, but these cases are exceptional. The other forms of acute myelogeous leukemia (AML), with the exception of acute progranulocytic leukemia (APL), remain resistant to therapy. APL is a unique disorder and is often associated with catastrophic bleeding disorder. However, several years ago it was discovered in China that a drug known as retinoic acid caused the leukemic promyelocytes to mature and this compound produced excellent remissions, but only for APL. It does not cause remissions in other forms of AML.

Recipes for Success

In the mid-1960s, many more treatment options became available to us. Vincent DeVita and his associates at the National Cancer Institute developed a program of combined chemotherapy called MOPP. This consisted of NH_2 (Mustogen), Oncovin (vincristine), Procarbazine and prednisone. Individually these drugs were not very effective, but, when combined, they worked on a deeper level with better results. When administered to patients with Hodgkin's disease, MOPP produced striking and prolonged remissions. Fever disappeared and large lymph node masses dramatically regressed; eventually MOPP produced 80% remissions. However, MOPP was not effective in other hematologic malignancies and it was realized that this approach was not the answer to treatment of leukemia and other malignancies. Nevertheless, the success of MOPP encouraged investigators to attempt to combine chemotherapeutic drugs in such a fashion that the malignant cells were attacked at several levels of metabolic activity. While no cures were obtained, over the years, more remissions occurred and life was prolonged in 70 to 80% of AML cases.

In 1963 or 1964 Sydney Farber's assistant, Tom Hall, asked if we would like to collaborate. They were treating children with combinations of chemotherapy, and thought we might want to try it on adults. Together we started a new form of chemotherapy program using drug combinations.

Aggressive chemotherapy programs were not universally approved. The strength of the drugs was a double-edged sword: if we didn't kill the tumor, we killed the patient. Many doctors felt this was indefensible, and editorials abounded, calling us "hawks." My feeling, and that of others like me, was that these drugs seemed the most promising and offered the most hope. We couldn't just sit back and wait for the development of some magic bullet; we had to take steps right away. We knew the alternative therapies would not provide remissions. Many of our patients agreed with us, and were willing to take the chance. In the end, it was the patients who made the decision which protocol to follow.

Among the more outspoken opponents were two preeminent American hematologists, Bill Dameshek and Bill Crosby. In 1966, during the annual meetings at Atlantic

City of the Old Turks and the Young Turks, a symposium on chemotherapy was sponsored by a loosely-organized group called the Blood Club. The panel of speakers included Dr. Dameshek as moderator, Jim Holland, George Brecher, Emil Frei, Wayne Rundles, and myself. Dr. Dameshek was a very caustic critic and enjoyed discomforting his opponents. The evening debate became particularly heated and Dr. Dameshek lashed out at those he called "hawks". When it came to be my turn to speak, I sought to defuse the tension and prefixed my remarks by saying we had spent the evening divided between the "hawks" and the "doves" but that it was a distinction to have the "bald eagle" of American hematology moderate the meeting. This greatly amused the large audience but infuriated the bald Dr. Dameshek.

Chapter Seven

LEGAL FALLOUT

AS A MEMBER of the U.S. Armed Forces Medical Committee, I was occasionally called upon to pay visits to various service establishments. One afternoon, I received a call and was told to report to Washington the next morning. This was unusually short notice; nevertheless it did not seem particularly out of the ordinary. From Washington I was flown, along with a group of doctors, to an airfield just outside Houston. We arrived late afternoon, and were bused to a large prairie. There, in the twilight, we were confronted with thousands of flickering lights stretching far into the night. Ambulances, hearses and trucks raced past us. There were large, company-sized tents set up, and rows and rows of "streets" staked and roped off into squares. As we walked along, we began to see signs hanging from the ropes of the squares. These were triage areas, and the signs, row after row of them, said simply, "Nothing to be done." It dawned on us then that we were seeing the effects of a mock attack. We learned the details at a briefing the next morning. The area was a near miss on Houston by a 50-megeton H-bomb. There were one million casualties. It staggered the imagination. All I could think of were those pathetic, hand-lettered signs. It chilled my blood.

As nuclear reactors began to be built throughout the United States, the Department of Energy formulated regulations to limit exposure to ionizing radiation. Committees were established to develop standards to govern the amount of exposure permitted. Because I was now known as an authority on radiation effects, I was asked by the government to act as an expert witness in a number of cases involving individuals exposed to ionizing radiation. Those cases dragged on for years, and continue to this day.

Expert Witness

One case involved a worker in an atomic energy plant whose job was to clean out the traps of the reactor complex. The man had developed acute myelogenous leukemia and had had considerable exposure (though not quantified) to radioactive material. I advised the company to settle without delay, which they did. Another case was not so straightforward. The patient, a union representative of MIT's building maintenance group, had a well-established diagnosis of acute leukemia. He worked in an infra-red laboratory. Shortly before his diagnosis, a spill of low level radioactive material had occurred two floors below the infra-red lab.

The timing of the spill and the diagnosis was simply coincidence, but to a public already primed with misinformation about the dangers of radioactive material, it seemed like a de facto case of cause and effect. I reviewed the information, and told his physician at MIT that there was no possible relationship between the man's leukemia and radiation exposure. Nevertheless, the insurance company settled the case. This was a tacit admission that the man's leukemia was radiation induced, which it was not, and a dangerous precedent had been set.

In 1963, a suit for $500,000 was brought against the Union Carbide Company in Oak Ridge, Tennessee on behalf of three workers claiming to have malignancies due to radiation exposure. The suit was presented on behalf of the workers by their union. During World War II, Union Carbide had been under contract with the government to produce plutonium for the manufacture of atomic bombs. Along with Dr. Leonard Hamilton, a world-renowned hematologist and radiation biologist from Sloan-Kettering, I was asked to help defend Union Carbide.

When I reviewed the cases, I found one patient had a diagnosis of chronic lymphatic leukemia, and the second had a case of Hodgkin's disease, neither of which was known to be induced by ionizing radiation. The third and last patient had a case of acute leukemia, but the radiation dose was too low to have caused it. Dr. Hamilton and I agreed that not one of the three diseases could be attributed to radiation exposure. The presiding Federal Court judge agreed and the case was dismissed.

A Bad Case of Bad Press

Over the following years I was engaged as an expert witness in a variety of cases. In every case, the doses of radiation were very low and all of the claims were dismissed. I'd made up my mind that I would not testify in any case where there was even a slight chance radiation doses were above acceptable levels. But the reality was that there were very few opportunities for the public to be exposed to high doses of ionizing radiation, other than in the instance of nuclear accident or a mishap during therapeutic radiation.

Unfortunately, scientific and medical press articles appeared which exaggerated out of all proportion the damages of radioactivity. The staid *New England Journal of Medicine* published an article by Lyons, a pediatrician, which claimed that part of Utah, as a result of fall-out from nuclear testing, had been heavily contaminated and had raised the incidence of childhood leukemia. Many epidemiologists protested these findings, and later studies of Utah soil samples proved Lyons's findings incorrect. An even more damaging article appeared in the *Lancet*, a widely-read British medical journal. The article claimed workers involved in the manufacture of nuclear submarines in the Portsmouth Naval Shipyard had a higher death rate from multiple myeloma than those workers who did not work with the nuclear submarines. These conclusions were drawn from a review of employee death certificates, not actual patient examinations.

No U.S. medical journal would print the *Lancet* report, but the *Boston Globe*, a newspaper known at the time for its anti-nuclear views, did. In addition, they funded follow-up studies, which were also printed. This created some serious production problems at the Portsmouth shipyard, as you can imagine. Admiral Rickover was dragged in to the controversy. Fearing that the Department of Energy would be biased, politicians refused to allow them to review the study.

The Center for Disease Control in Atlanta, with no expertise in the field, was asked to repeat the study. The findings of the *Lancet* article were found to be incorrect. The *Boston Globe* did print this, but buried it on page twelve. This article, as well as numerous other ones, did extensive damage to the nuclear program, and were to a large part responsible for the misunderstanding, fear and hysteria surrounding the use of nuclear power. This fear was rampant, and pervaded even into the courtroom.

Taking a Stand

The Justice Department was frustrated by the fact that, case after case, totaling hundreds of thousands of dollars, was being decided against the government. Ralph Johnson, trial attorney for the Justice Department, came to see me at Brigham and Women's Hospital and asked if I could work under government contract as an expert witness for the number of cases pending trial. I refused, because I knew being "under contract" would ruin my credibility with a jury. I did, however, offer to act as witness for those cases in which I believed the plaintiffs were wrong.

Most of the cases against the government had no merit and were easily defended. However, there was a landmark case in 1986 which involved five plaintiffs who worked dismantling bomb sights in a plant in Wichita, Kansas. These plaintiffs had just won a suit against their employer for several million dollars, and were now alleging the U.S. government had been negligent in labeling the bomb sights.

I was part of a cadre of well-trained lawyers and experts in the field of nuclear physics that made up the government's defense team. We met in Wichita and carefully prepared for the trial.

The plaintiffs had enjoyed success after success and seemed unbeatable. One of their experts was Dr. John Gofman, a Ph.D. and M.D., and author of a book about the ill effects of ionizing radiation. He seemed more of an antinuclear activist than a scientist. Another expert for the plaintiff had been one of the foremost practitioners in the emerging field of radiation protection. He had been a pioneer, and had taught a great many of the present day experts, including some testifying for the U.S at this trial. The third person on their team was a graduate of the Harvard School of Public Health and was well-known for testifying against the U.S.

The Justice Department lawyers took the position that the best defense was a good offense. They challenged the experts repeatedly and were not intimidated by the credentials they presented. While on the stand, Dr. Gofman was pompous and condescending, quick to point out that he was a physician as well as a nuclear scientist, and espoused at length the famous physicists he had worked with. Our lawyers questioned the venerable Dr. Gofman's qualifications in medical practice, and it came out that the doctor did not practice medicine actively, had meager training, and had not been on the staff of any hospital for years.

When asked his opinion in the case of lower colon cancer in one of the plaintiffs, Dr. Gofman agreed that the external dose of radiation was low, but held firm to his claim that flakes of radioactive paint had been ingested, traveled down the bowel and concentrated in the crypts of the lower bowel. When asked how he knew the cancer was in the lower colon, he replied, "because the examining doctor palpated the mass." The lawyer quietly pointed out that the tumor could not be palpated from below. He then followed with a simple medical question: "Dr. Gofman, what is the length of the rectum?" Gofman replied, incorrectly, "3 or 4 inches." The lawyer countered that the anal canal was 8 inches long, thus requiring a pretty long finger to reach the tumor. Dr. Gofman's testimony was discredited, as was he.

Dr. Ralph Z. Morgan, the other "ringer" for the plaintiffs, had been a pioneer and an outstanding teacher in the field of radiation protection. This was readily admitted by the defense. But they pointed out that Dr. Morgan had developed a new career testifying for plaintiffs against the U.S. He also was quickly discredited, as were the remaining witnesses with even fewer credentials. Judge Patrick Kelly dismissed the suit against the government and, in an opinion published in the *Law Review*, stated that these two doctors had deliberately misled the court and should not be allowed to testify again in a federal court.

Many of the cases I was involved in were frivolous, and a waste of everyone's time. Nuclear energy, when controlled, was incredibly useful. But as much as I had been advocating for, and testifying about the benefits of nuclear energy, experiencing the mock attack on Houston showed me a side of it I prayed I would never see.

Chapter Eight

UNDER THE HOUSE CALLS

The Marshall Islands, 1962 and 1963

NOT ALL the exposed natives could come in for examinations, so we hiked to the outlying areas and carried out our examinations and obtained blood specimens in the field. We also had to travel to several nearby atolls in a small dory-like boat. The wind and the rushing tide made getting through the passes rather difficult, and we invariably arrived at our destinations soaking wet. On one trip we were accompanied by native doctors, and traveled with them in a small boat. No sooner were we out in open water than the boat capsized. Doctors and equipment were thrown into the water. Fortunately, the equipment had been carefully waterproofed and protected, and it was fine. The doctors, unfortunately, were not so carefully protected.

On March 11, 1954 the United States detonated the H-bomb "Bravo" over the Marshall Islands. The yield of this explosion was in the twenty megaton range. While the explosion was planned, the fallout was not. Usually in

March the prevailing winds blew to the west. However, for unknown meteorological reasons, on the day of the detonation the winds blew to the east and the debris from the pulverized Bikini Atoll formed a huge radioactive cloud that extended northeast over the Marshall Islands.

I participated in an on-going study of those Marshallese natives who had been exposed to fall-out from the explosion. Fortunately there were no natives on the northern islands where radioactivity from the fallout measured two to three thousand rads. But on the southern fringe of the cloud on the atolls of Alinginas, Rongelap and Rongerick, seventy to 100 miles east of Bikini, there were eighty-two natives and twenty-eight American service men who received an average of 175 rads from gamma emitting fallout. On Utirik atoll, 300 miles from Bikini, 157 natives received fourteen rads. There were beta radiation burns on some natives due to the radioactive dust deposited on the skin, but these burns were superficial and healed completely.

Within seventy-two hours of the detonation of Bravo, special US Naval teams were sent out and exposed individuals were evacuated to Kwajalein Island. A team of experts from the Naval Research Institute and the Naval Radiological Defense Laboratory were sent to Kwajalein to carry out intensive studies to evaluate the amount and characteristics of the radioactivity. After several months, the Utirik natives were allowed to return to their island. But Rongelap remained highly radioactive so the natives were moved to a temporary village on Marjuro.

By 1957, Rongelap atoll was considered safe for habitation and the people were transported back to their island where a new village had been constructed by workers from the Department of Energy. Subsequent annual surveys have been conducted and a series of reports published by E.P. Cronkite, V.P. Bond, C.L. Durham and R.A. Conard and co-workers.

Going Native

In February 1961 I was asked to participate in the study on the Marshallese and joined a team of five U.S. physicians, three laboratory technicians and one electronics expert. After being processed through U.S. Navy channels in Honolulu, we flew the remaining 2400 miles by Military Air Transportation to Kwajalein. This island was an important deep water port that was heavily defended by the Japanese during the Second World War. The island was 2.5 miles long and less than one-half mile wide. It consisted of a reef surrounded by more than 100 small atolls, and a lagoon sixty-six miles long and two miles wide. We approached the island at dawn, coming down out of the low clouds to the unexpected sight of buildings the size of a department store, some of which housed the missile station with its launch pad and array of radar and computer installations.

We were put up in the Navy BOQ and the next day were loaded aboard the Ron Anmin, a 250-ton inter-island ship, for the 150-mile trip to Rongelap. When we got out of the lee of the islands the west wind kicked up huge waves and we plunged up and down, with the sea breaking over the ship. I stayed in my bunk, bracing myself against the wall and managed to weather it without much trouble. We reached the Pass into the Rongelap lagoon and were greeted with the lovely sight of a long, curving shore with palm trees waving in the background. Since there was no dock everything had to be moved ashore in small boats, including us. We all pitched in and eventually most of our equipment and supplies were off-loaded. The Navy ferried the generator for our electricity and fifty drums of water and eight drums of gasoline were bulldozed up to our campsite. The tent was set up on the wooden floor Navy carpenters had already built in preparation for our arrival. We slept on cots and with the sides of the tent rolled up it was quite comfortable. We also rented several native shacks to use as kitchen, laboratory and examining rooms. The natives were friendly. Many of them spoke English and had worked for the Missile site people. We had two native "doctors" who proved to be very useful to us.

Physicians in the Field

Our mission on Rongelap was to examine 240 Marshallese. These included exposed adults and children and children born to exposed parents. We also looked at a comparison population of unexposed natives. One excursion to see a native brought me out to see a very old man, said to be about ninety, who lived alone in his U.S. built hut. Actually, for reasons unknown to me, he chose to live underneath his hut, so that's where I had to go to examine him. An awkward situation under the best of circumstances was made all the more complicated by the arrival of a flock of hens, followed by a herd of small pigs. I called it my "under-the-house" visit.

On March 22, the Ron Anmin returned to Rongelap to

bring us back to Kwajalein. On the way there we received a radio message to divert to the island of Panope in the Carolinas to examine a young native who had been exposed on Rongelap. The Navy flew us 400 miles west to this beautiful tropical island, abundant with lush fruits and vegetation. We were royally treated by the District Administrator of the Trust Territory, Maynard Neas. After examining the child we returned to Kwajalein. We packed up our specimens and exam results and on March 26 left for Honolulu, then home to decipher our results.

Medical Findings

There were no significant findings in our studies of the exposed adult Marshallese. The somewhat lowered white cell counts noted by other physicians on earlier visits had returned to normal. We had attempted to obtain bone marrow on ten different exposed natives to carry out chromosome studies. In a few cases, we did note abnormal chromosomes, but due to the heat and humidity the chromosome preparations were not very successful, so the results were inconclusive.

One year later, in March 1963, I came back for another visit to the Marshall Islands. Not much had changed in a year, but when we arrived on Kwajalein we were dismayed to learn that disaster had struck the natives in the form of an epidemic paralytic poliomyelitis. About eighty children and a few young adults were affected, and the Navy ferried them down to Majuro where there was a converted Naval Station Hospital. We flew there to see if we could help but there was little we could do. Three children had paralysis

of the respiratory muscles but the hospital had only one
iron lung (respirator). The doctors tried valiantly to rotate
the three children on the respirator, but all three died. The
Navy did all it could, and the Red Cross and other agencies
pitched in and soon things greatly improved. Apparently
no one thought to give the Salk vaccine to the Marshallese,
although the vaccine had been available. The Trust Territory was a peculiar establishment and the natives just fell
through the cracks.

Near Miss

After some delay, we were flown back to Rongelap, with
the intent to fly from there to Utirik Atoll. When we
departed from Rongelap the plane was pretty heavily
loaded. It was nerve-racking to see the pilot of the PBY
struggle to get it into the air. We barely missed the reef,
and were just beginning to relax when our sighs of relief
were cut short by the explosion of the port engine. Smoke
and flames shot out and the Navy crewman came dashing
down the aisle shouting for us to put on our Mae Wests
and to pull out our shark repellent. In a feeling that was
becoming all too familiar, I found myself in an airplane,
making preparations not to be. The life jacket went on
quickly, experienced as I now was, and I held the shark
repellent with a death grip. Fortunately, neither were necessary. The fire was put out quickly and we hobbled back
to Kwajalein on one engine. I swore I would never fly
again. But as soon as we landed we were rushed to another
plane and the journey began all over again. I found myself

reviewing my salary in my head, and, while I don't remember what the exact sum was, I do know that at the time I was feeling it was not nearly enough.

Lost

We made it to Utirik, a beautiful, palm-tree covered island with its own water supply. Before getting to work, I decided to take a walk around the island, and Leo Meyer, a pathologist on our team, went with me. Utirik was small, only about a mile wide. It seemed a simple enough plan to walk around it. We started out along the lagoon, and after walking about 1/2 hour and collecting a few shells and glass fishing balls, started back. Or thought we'd started back. We didn't seem to be making any progress toward camp. I pointed out to Leo that we'd passed the same broken palm tree three times. Leo sat down and started to laugh and stated the obvious: "Moloney, we are lost!"

Ten years ago, when Leo was first asked to join this expedition, he was not sure if he wanted to go. So he went to consult with Professor Krumbhaar, the doyen of pathologists. Krumbhaar, who had published a history of pathology in 1937, was professor of pathology at the University of Pennsylvania. He asked Leo if the natives were friendly. Leo knew enough to assure the professor they were. With that, Professor Krumbhaar leaned back in his chair and let loose his only other concern: "Leo, did you ever hear of a Jewish explorer?" We laughed as Leo recounted the story, and whether by happenstance or design, I took the lead and found a trail that led us back to camp.

Back to Work

On Uterik we examined 157 exposed Marshallese. By the time the radioactive cloud had reached Utirik, the radioactivity had greatly decreased. It was estimated that the natives received about fifteen rads from the fallout. A few years later, pediatricians found thyroid nodules in the Rongelap and Utirik children. Some were benign thyroid tumors, others were malignant. Fortunately surgical removal (some of it performed in Boston) cured all these patients. It was concluded that radioactive ash had fallen into the open cisterns, the islands' only water supply. When ingested, it traveled to the thyroid gland and concentrated in that organ. Children were particularly susceptible. It was determined that while the major part of the radioactivity was due to I-131, shorter lived isotopes of iodine had also been created and caused high doses of radiation locally in the thyroid glands. Today, similar problems are being encountered as a result of fallout from the Chernobyl accident.

This visit to Utirik was my last assignment. I have often thought about the Marshallese and their unfortunate life circumstances. Following World War I and German supervision, they were entrusted to the Japanese. The Japanese taught them how to grow crops and employed them in the construction of military bases, especially on Kwajalein Atoll. This island was subject to some ferocious fighting before it fell to the U.S. marines and army units. We then used Einewetock and Bikini Atolls for our thermonuclear weapons testing, displacing the natives to other islands to do so. Following this, as part of our Pacific defenses, we established powerful radar with inter-continental missile sites and other facilities on the islands. These installations caused further disruption of the Marshallese natives, and the final insult was the fallout from Bravo.

The United States has been roundly criticized for its role in these events. However, very real efforts were made to aid the Marshallese and it is too often forgotten that during the Cold War, the U.S. was in a race with Russia to produce the H-Bomb. Widespread misunderstanding of the dangers of radiation, supported by the media and sensationalized by the cinema, made Americans unnecessarily fearful, and that fear was exacerbated when British spies, such as Klaus Fuchs, Kim Philby, MacLean, as well as those at Cambridge University under the supervision of Sir Anthony Blount, infiltrated our nuclear laboratories and turned over to the Russians all our nuclear weapon secrets. Unfortunately, the power and influence of people like Joseph McCarthy made it difficult to defend efforts in this country and in England to uncover and combat these individuals. In the long run, as Americans, we did what we had to do, and I for one do not think we should be ashamed of our efforts.

While involving only a relatively small population, the impact of "Bravo" furnished some frightening observations. The radioactive cloud stretched for 300 miles. Heaviest fallout was two to three thousand rads, with residual radiation that persisted for years. These sobering results were made available to the Russians, as well as the U.S. and our allies, and no doubt had a significant influence against the use of nuclear weapons.

Chapter Nine

COWBARNS AND CATHOUSES

WE ONLY GAVE money to worthwhile applicants, and there were some years when we didn't give out all the allotted funds, simply because there were not enough qualified applicants. I remember being chastised by Father Mike Walsh, the head of the Boston College pre-med program. He challenged me for rejecting their grant applications year after year. I pointed out that they were consistently bad. "Well, that's your fault," he told me. It was up to me, apparently, to show them how to write a proper grant application. So there I was, on yet another committee.

I joined the American Cancer Society (ACS) in 1961, motivated primarily by hopes of attaining some grant money. While my motives may not have been entirely altruistic, I grew to love this organization. The ACS is the largest and probably one of the most influential private organizations in the world. Founded in 1945, it had its beginning in Boston and New York, and membership was made up of chiefly surgeons. Prior to 1960, there were few methods of treatment for cancer except surgery and radiation therapy. Cancer was considered, with few exceptions, to be universally fatal and few doctors other than surgeons played an active role in the treatment of the disease. It was undertstandable that the ACS would originally be comprised mostly of surgeons.

Cancer Comes Out of the Closet

As late as the early 1950s, the public at large was not aware of cancer. There was such a stigma attached to it that no one would admit they had the disease. It was the tobacco link to cancer that finally broke the story. Epidemiologists and chest surgeons finally began to recognize the role of cigarette smoking as a cause of cancer of the lung. Soon great efforts were made to eliminate smoking and the public became informed about cancer of the lung. Other efforts at cancer detection and education included the Papanicolaou smear to detect cancer of the cervix, and women were instructed in breast examination techniques. The ACS played an increasingly prominent role in these areas. Although not connected with any governmental agencies, this strictly volunteer organization rapidly surged to the top of the cancer detection and prevention fields. Membership was open to all. Half of the volunteers were physicians or other health professionals while the other half was made up of lay people.

The American Cancer Society is composed of some fifty or more chapters, usually one for each state. In some areas, such as Boston, New York, Philadelphia, St. Louis, New Orleans, and other noted medical centers, a tremendous amount of talent is available to the Society. The West Coast chapters prevailed upon famous actors and actresses to raise large amounts of money and create increasing interest in the problem of cancer. Since one out of four individuals dies of some form of malignancy, it was a cause which drew a great deal of interest, especially as it began to be publicized that prominent and well-respected people had died of cancer. Cancer of the lung, especially, gained wide notoriety among the Hollywood set.

Granting Grants

Shortly after joining the ACS, I was made Chairman of the Research Committee. In the early days, funds were very limited and research applications were pretty pedestrian, e.g., comparative studies on the efficiency of various surgical methods for treating breast cancer or similar projects. Though our funds were limited, we were determined that the money would be well spent. Grant proposals were reviewed by peers, and while the grants were small—never more than $10,000, and usually in the $2,000-$3,000 range—they primed the pump for the work of several local doctors, myself among them. As I published and became better known, I was able to obtain the larger NIH and AEC grants.

As time went on, along with the rapid developments in biochemistry, genetics, viral oncology, and other basic sciences, grant applications became much more sophisticated with requests coming in for larger sums of money than we were accustomed to giving out. It became clear we'd need help in reviewing this new breed of requests, and fortunately, we were able to recruit outstanding people from the hospitals and medical schools to serve on the ACS research committee.

ACS Makes Its Mark

Hitherto, cancer research was almost exclusively in the hands of young physicians and surgeons. However, with the extraordinary explosion of knowledge in the 60s and 70s, young Ph.D.s began to take over the field, increasingly so in cytogenetics, molecular biology, immunology, and other basic areas. The need for specially trained individuals who would remain on a full-time basis created a demand for research fellowships and professorships. The NIH provided the bulk of these but, beginning in the 1960s, the ACS developed programs ranging from the undergraduate level to full professorships. These were funded for the most part by NIH, but in some areas, such as Boston, generous donors provided funds for special research fellowships and professorships. One of the earliest programs was supported by a three million dollar grant from the estate of Peter Fuller.

Although Boston, with its three medical schools, MIT and other outstanding institutions, had an enviable reputation in the medical field, a serious deficiency was the lack of excellent radiation therapy facilities. The ACS, through its research committees, decided that one million dollars each from the Fuller grant should be awarded to Harvard, Tufts, and Boston University Medical School. This enabled Samuel Hellman to be appointed Chief of Radiation Oncology at Harvard Medical School in 1968. His department included the then Peter Bent Brigham Hospital, the Children's Hospital, and the newly organized Children's Cancer Research Foundation (later known as the Dana-Farber Cancer Research Foundation) and the Beth Israel Hospital. Sam Hellman was an outstanding doctor and radiotherapist. He built up a superior department, trained numerous professors in radiation therapy, and co-authored several classical textbooks on cancer therapy. Dr. Hellman became the first Peter Fuller Professor.

At BU Medical School, it was decided to build and staff a Betatron unit. This was a unique unit and was headed by a Fuller Professor. Meanwhile, an effort was made to encourage medical students and young physicians to become involved with medical research. A junior Peter Fuller Fellowship was designed to support fellows in the early years of training; later on with the generous support of the Betty Lea Stone Fellowship Foundation, the ACS was able to establish part-time fellowships for pre-med students. Each medical school, including the newly opened University of Massachusetts Medical School, was allotted one fellowship. This program, which was initially organized by a committee consisting of Harold Amos, Paul Christopher, Hughes Rysner and myself, continues to be highly successful.

Great strides have been made in raising large amounts of money for the fight against cancer, not only on a state level, but also nationally. Progress has been made in educating the public about cancer. Moreover, a variety of special needs, e.g., care of osteotomies, rehabilitation, breast prosthesis, and other supportive activities have been actively pursued. In all these activities, the Massachusetts Division and the National society have played a major role.

As potent chemotherapy and radiation therapy progressed, the need for skilled and well-trained nurses, nurse practitioners, and nurse assistants became essential. The concept of the oncology nurse was developed, although not always welcomed by some older members of the medical profession. The awarding of professorships and assistant professorships in oncology nursing was actively supported by the ACS. Much the same can be said about developments in the field of Social Service.

President of Massachusetts ACS

As a physician and one chiefly interested in medical research, I did not pay much attention to other activities of the American Cancer Society. Nor did I fully appreciate the unselfish contributions, in time and money, that were made by the volunteers and many of the staff. After becoming President of the Massachusetts division of the American Cancer Society in 1968, I became well acquainted with the broad range of ACS activities. Paul Christopher was assistant to the Executive Secretary, James Lavin, when I joined the ACS. Jim became ill and died shortly thereafter and Paul became Executive Secretary. A better choice could not have been made. Paul had a disingenuous manner which concealed a very tough character. He was particularly adept at involving his friends and associates in various plans for the Society. My wife, Jo, Alice Christopher, and Paul became close friends and we often traveled together to New York City for the annual meetings.

To illustrate Paul's methods, he was particularly interested in promoting a higher status for oncology nurses, and wanted specifically to establish a professorship in oncology nursing. Paul asked me to propose this to the National Executive Secretary, Lane Adams. I always believed that Mr. Adams felt challenged by the Massachusetts Division and did not particularly like us as a group. Nonetheless, Paul led me to his office in New York, pushed me in before him, and told Adams I wanted to talk to him about the oncology nurses. This did not particularly please Lane and his lack of enthusiasm got my back up. So, I made an impassioned demand and Paul and I stalked out of his office. Much to the gratification of the nurses, the proposal to create professorships for oncology nurses was accepted.

On another occasion, we got into a row with the then Dean of Harvard Medical School. After the grant of a million dollars to Harvard for an oncology professorship, Peter Fuller, who had remained active on the American Cancer Society's Board of Directors, was displeased because he was informed that, after a year, the individual to whom the grant was awarded had not taken up the mouse research he was hired to do. Peter Fuller spoke to Paul, and Paul informed me that we had to see the Dean and get the matter straightened out. The Dean was not hostile to our visit but he was plainly not impressed with our complaint.

Paul then told the Dean that Mr. Fuller was not pleased, and the Dean replied that Harvard was not in the habit of accepting directions for its activities. Paul and I pointed out then that we would tell Mr. Fuller to withdraw the million dollars if the situation was not remedied. As a result, the grant was shifted to a very active and outstanding cancer researcher and other funds were apparently found for the

prior recipient. Deans, even from Harvard, did not intimi-
date Paul Christopher. It was a pleasure to work with Paul
and his excellent and loyal staff. He retired in 1987 but
continued on as an advisor and friend of the ACS.

Volunteers Extraordinaire

It is difficult to single out individuals from the very large
group of excellent volunteers, but two stand out in my
mind: Mrs. Robert Stone, Betty Lea to her friends, and
Stanley Shmiskis. Betty Lea started out before World War
I working as a college volunteer at the famous Huntington
Memorial Hospital for Cancer Research. Betty Lea came
from a wealthy and aristocratic background, but she was
one of the most democratic and ecumenical people I ever
knew. When the ACS was organized, she joined the Board
of Directors and was an active and articulate member.

On the occasion of her eightieth birthday, friends and
relations established a research fund in her honor. Mrs.
Stone asked Paul Christopher to form a small committee
to help determine what to do with the fund. Paul requested
that Harold Amos, who was a professor of microbiology
at Harvard, and myself meet the Stone family to discuss
the matter. Robert Stone was still alive at the time and we
drove out to his estate in Dedham and met with Mr. and
Mrs. Stone and their sons. We recognized that there was a
critical situation developing in medical research, i.e., increasingly young physicians were not going into basic
research. Harold Amos suggested that we establish a Stone
Junior Research Fellowship at each of the four Massachusetts medical Schools. These fellowships would be offered

to successful candidates who were in their first year of medicine.

It was pointed out that in later years of medical school, there would be no opportunity to spend a summer doing research. A proctor would arrange that the fellow be involved with an ongoing cancer research project and interact actively with older colleagues. The Stone family agreed with this plan, and the ACS, through its Massachusetts Division, made the necessary arrangements. This Junior Research Fellowship has proven to be a very successful program and has attracted many young scientists to the field of medical research. Mrs. Robert Stone is now well over ninety but she continues to have an active interest in young people and in the American Cancer Society.

The other volunteer who has had an exceptional impact, not only in Massachusetts but on a national and world-wide level, is Stanley Shmiskis. He is a very successful businessman and realtor in Lynn, Massachusetts, and became a member of the Board of Trustees of the Massachusetts Division. Stanley not only made his own major financial gifts to the ACS, but, more importantly, he became a very industrious and important committee member. With his professional knowledge of the real estate business, Stanley was able to offer important advice and council on many occasions regarding purchase or evaluation of property.

Stanley was made a member of the National Board of Directors and then became its Secretary. He was instrumental in establishing the American Cancer Society Foundation. This organization has already raised considerable funds and has earned an international reputation. It includes in its membership and Board of Trustees many of the most prestigious individuals in the American professional and business world. Paul Christopher, Betty Lee Stone and Stanley Shmiskis epitomize the dedicated spirit of the ACS volunteers and ACS staff and explain the amazing success of this organization.

The SALES Committee

Another organization important to my career was the SALES (Special Animal Leukemia Etiology Studies) Committee. Its establishment was a natural follow-up to a series of important discoveries. I was honored when my old friend and limo partner, John Moloney, called to ask if I'd join him as a member of this prestigious committee.

The period from 1948 to the present has witnessed unprecedented progress in modern medical science. In 1951, Watson and Crick described the double helix structure of DNA. Oncogenic viruses were rediscovered and, with the electron microscope, typical particles became visible to the eye, chiefly due to the pioneering work of Leon Dmochowski and Joseph Beard in 1954. Once C particles or viruses were recognized under electron microscopy, studies were carried out in all parts of tissues and body fluids. In 1964, John Moloney described three new retroviruses in mouse leukemias and sarcomas. Eric Gross, who had been demonstrating cell-free passage of mouse leukemia since 1951, was finally vindicated. In 1964, C particles were discovered in cow's milk and in chickens.

These discoveries were noted by the press, and articles in the *New York Times* publicized the findings. Immediately, politicians began to demand that the government investigate the situation. As a result, a special appropriation of ten million dollars was made available to the National Cancer Institute to set up a viral oncology program. The SALES committee was established as a medium to organize it. A number of young virologists, some of whom had been working on poliomyelitis, were recruited into the program, and John Moloney was hired as Director.

Only two of the twelve committee members were M.D.s; the others were Ph.D.'s in virology, every one of whom had discovered their own, non-baloney virus. The committee met in Washington every four to six months and reviewed grant applications and contracts. In general, the calibre of the proposals we received was quite high. On one occasion, we were arguing over whether to fund cattle research at the University of California at Davis, or cat leukemia research in Syracuse. This meeting, as well as most others, got quite heated. There was screaming across the table as each doctor tried to get their view across. Everyone had their own opinion as to which program was more important: cowbarns in Davis or cathouses in Syracuse. It was so loud no one could hear anything. My contribution was to yell even louder at everyone to sit down and calm down, all the while rapping on the table like Kruschev in order to get their attention.

By the end of the 1970s, interest in finding a human leukemia virus had waned, and molecular biologists took over the field. These biologists could barely hide their disdain for clinicians and virologists. "I have no interest in patients," a well-known biologist proudly remarked. In truth, they didn't so much take over the field as wrest it away. The discovery by Watson and Crick of the structure of DNA paved the way for the flood of investigations which led to Baltimore's and Temin's discovery of reverse transcriptase. Subsequent research developed the concept of the oncogene and proto-oncogenes. With the cloning of oncogenes it then became possible to recognize the role of the ras oncogene and the suppressor genes: APC, DCC and p53. As Robert Weinberg has pointed out, the occurrence of malignancy is not a sudden change, but is the result of a series of mutations activating events along with loss of suppressor gene activity. These discoveries have not fully solved the problem of cancer, but have created new and innovative pathways for investigation.

I served on the SALES Committee until 1970. The budget rose each year until it reached seventy million dollars in 1978, the year the committee disbanded. There were many criticisms of this viral oncology program, some not justified. However, while the ultimate goal of the program was not achieved, a great deal of good was derived from work done under auspices of the SALES Committee. Some of the programs supported seemed esoteric at the time, but later, even one of its strongest critics, Robert Weinstein, admitted that several important contributions had been made. In fact, Robert Gallo has acknowledged the SALES Committee for supporting some of his work which led ultimately to the identification of the AIDS virus, HTLV-1.

Chapter Ten

CHEMOTHERAPY IN THE CORRIDORS

1962–1973

MY OFFICE at the Brigham consisted of one small office with one exam room, and a waiting room shared with Dr. Richard Wilson. Dick was a tall, bluff fellow and an excellent surgeon. His secretary was very prim. She was not at all happy when my practice took off and my patients began to crowd the small waiting room. If Dick's exam room was empty we would try to sneak overflow patients in there, but were often caught by the secretary who would summarily throw us out.

As the turbulent 1960s progressed I became increasingly disillusioned at Boston City Hospital. Once insurance companies started paying for care, patients migrated to the more upscale institutions such as the Brigham and the Faulkner. Those patients who did continue on with us came mostly from nearby predominantly black and Hispanic neighborhoods. Activists within both these groups influenced appointments to the professional staff, and an overall decline began. The important people at BCH started to leave. Franz Ingelfinger, Chief of Medicine at Boston University and editor of *The New England Journal of Medicine* was one of several leaving BCH. "The rats are leaving the ship," he said to me. And he was right. Qualified doctors left in droves. I, however, stayed on. I was in my late 50s by then and felt too old to start over someplace new.

A Face Lift

Besides, things for me really weren't all that bad. In 1959 and again in 1962, Dr. Sydney Farber helped me obtain a $150,000 institutional grant. This enabled Tufts, for the first time, to have adequate teaching and research quarters in a wing of the original hospital. The building we occupied was built in 1864, and at the time was considered one of the finest examples of hospital architecture in the country. Hospital ceilings soared thirty feet, and great windows reached from ceiling to floor. Many famous visitors had toured this wing, among them Florence Nightingale. But in spite of this pedigree, the grand old building was falling apart.

With the grant money and a very cooperative superintendent, John Conlin, we were able to reconstruct three floors of the building. The top floor was for Dr. Maurice Segal and the Lung Station; the middle floor was for cardiology laboratories and facilities; and the first floor for the Tufts Hematology Laboratory. Here we built chemistry and hematology laboratories, examining rooms, a waiting room, and offices. It was really an elegant place and we were all delighted with it. I convinced Conlin to invest

$80,000 of the hospital money to fix up the basement, thereby giving us extra space for a large conference room and a locker room for the Tufts medical students.

These renovations did much to improve the quality of life for the hematologists at BCH, but I continued to be frustrated by the lack of inpatient facilities. The open wards persisted, with the few private rooms utilized for dying or disturbed patients. I had no choice but to admit my patients to the Faulkner Hospital. I was dissatisfied with this arrangement, but knew it would not change. Tufts continued to focus its attention and resources on developing the New England Medical Center. So even though BCH provided most of the Tufts teaching beds, little support was forthcoming from Tufts. I was resigned to the situation.

A New Life

Unexpectedly, in 1966 I was approached by members of the search committee from the Peter Bent Brigham Hospital. Dr. Frank Gardner had resigned in 1965 as Chief of Hematology and no one had been appointed in his place. They needed a hematologist to help with their pioneering work on bone marrow transplants and renal transplants. I was flattered and overjoyed when they asked if I'd be interested in the job; the offer seemed to me to be a near miracle. Behind it, I knew, was the influence of Sidney Farber and several outstanding young physicians on the Peter Bent Brigham Hospital staff. These younger fellows knew me chiefly through my efforts with the American Federation for Clinical Research. I gratefully accepted the dual position of Chief of the Hematology Division at

PBBH and Chief of Hematology at the Jimmy Fund, associated with the Children's Hospital.

With Dr. Farber's support, I was able to take David Rosenthal with me as a Senior Fellow. David was a Godsend. He was an excellent clinician and teacher, and gave a lot of attention to the house staff, patients and students. He was tireless; the hardest worker I ever knew. I couldn't have done anything without him. While I was tied up with daily rounds, David saw all our patients. He also indulged my fertile imagination, and would work with me on a myriad of experiments. We published several papers together.

All our patients, with a few exceptions, would first be seen and examined by the Hematology fellow or medical resident. Then David or myself would see the patient, go over the findings and decide which laboratory studies should be carried out. A high percentage of cases required bone marrow examination; the aspiration or biopsy was done by the fellow or resident, supervised usually by David or myself. By this time, special marrow biopsy needles were available, which made obtaining specimens much easier.

David and I used to sit in the lab in the afternoon looking at the bone marrow specimens through the two-headed scope. As it became known that David and I could be found looking at slides every afternoon, the house staff began wandering by asking if they could participate. I could see it was time to dust off my old teaching kit from BCH. The William Moloney Bone Marrow Course was as popular at the Brigham as it had been at Boston City. We often had a large backlog of people waiting to take it.

No such course had ever been offered at the Peter Bent
Brigham Hospital. Doctors had their own patients and were
very territorial about them. They ran the hospital like a
series of dukedoms. I remember consulting on a case of
multiple myeloma at the Brigham in 1966, before I joined
as full-time staff. I took a bone marrow specimen and asked
the intern if he'd like to look at it with me. His jaw
dropped. He'd never before been allowed to do such a
thing. The doctor in charge of the case was furious with
me, and said I'd never be asked to consult there again. This
type of attitude always astonished me. What was the point
in being there if not to cure and to teach?

And a New Lab

The Peter Bent Brigham Hospital was in all respects different from Boston City Hospital. They doubled my salary,
gave me a $100,000 life insurance policy, paid my Blue
Cross and Blue Shield fees, and put me in contact with a
financial advisor who started me on an investment and
retirement plan. Yet, surprisingly, their lab conditions were
awful. I toured the hematology laboratory prior to accepting the position and was shocked by the slovenly habits of
the technicians: they wore dirty lab coats, had out of date
laboratory equipment, and had appalling sanitary conditions. Urine and stool examinations were performed at the
same bench used for blood studies! I was astonished. The
interns and residents I spoke with viewed the hematology
lab with disdain, and admitted that any results coming from
there were not considered reliable.

I gave Dr. Thorn a "behind the scenes" tour of this lab,

after which he readily agreed to reconstruct and enlarge it. I was able to throw out the antiquated research equipment and obtain space for special laboratory procedures. I then set about upgrading the lab staff. Fortunately the lady who "ran" the laboratory quickly resigned, and I was able to hire a fine, well-trained chief technician who was a real disciplinarian. She hand-picked new staff and the whole operation was greatly upgraded.

We began to see an increasing number of cases of leukemia, as well as Hodgkin's disease, malignant lymphoma, and multiple myeloma. For these latter disorders, radiation therapy was the treatment of choice; however, the PBBH had a very poor radiation therapy department. Fortunately, the year after I arrived a new department was created with Dr. Samuel Hellman as Chief of Radiation Therapy. Newer high voltage X-ray machines became available and the Brigham rapidly surged to the top in the field of radiation oncology.

Radiation vs. Oncology

Sam proved to be a superb radiation therapist and a wonderful teacher. Many of Sam Hellman's fellows went on to become professors and chairmen of radiation oncology departments. One in particular was outstanding. Joel Greenburger came to me as a third year Harvard Medical student. He became interested in working on enzymes called lysozymes which were found in mononuclear cells, and took off one year from medical school to work on some interesting experiments with these enzymes. Joel spent two years at Boston City Hospital in medicine, then decided he wanted to go into viral oncology. He went to the National Institute of Health as a research fellow, where he worked with mice for two years; but, disillusioned by the aggressive, ambitious people in Washington, he then took a fellowship in radiation therapy with Sam Hellman and was able to combine the radiation therapy training and his cell culture work. Joel became Chief of Radiation Therapy at the University of Massachusetts and after a few years accepted the post of Professor of Radiation Oncology at the University of Pittsburgh Medical School. I continued to work with Joel for several years and was a co-author on a number of his papers.

Joint rounds occurred on a weekly basis at the Brigham. Discussions of case management could get rather heated as each side advocated their preferred protocol. Dr. Hellman, understandably, was in favor of radiation. But great strides were being made with chemotherapy and many doctors were beginning to feel this was the preferred treatment. The most vocal advocate for chemotherapy was George Canellos from the Dana-Farber Cancer group. George liked to stir things up and the noise at those meetings often reached ear-shattering levels.

I had presented a paper at the 1966 Atlantic City Hematology Conference illustrating the success we were having with the multiple-agent chemotherapy combination we called VAMP. Once we were established at PBBH, David and I made some adjustments to this combination therapy. By then, newer agents were available and we combined AraC with daunarubicin. The combination proved to be very effective, and is still used today. While there was no question about the effectiveness of aggressive chemotherapy, the newer agents were difficult to work with. If DNA got out of the vein on injection a severe local reaction resulted, leading at times to necrosis and ulceration. And many patients developed severe complications from the drugs: bleeding disorders, mucosal ulcerations, cardiac disorders and infectious diseases were the most common.

Administering the drugs required expertise across many areas of medicine, as well as the resources of a well-equipped hospital. The chemotherapy unit evolved as David and our fellows worked to put in place all the equipment and expertise we felt necessary to administer the drugs. I remember going to the blood bank and asking for twenty units of platelets. The head of the bank was appalled and refused my request, saying it simply wasn't possible for him to give me so much. I knew we'd have an ongoing need for a well-stocked blood bank, and since I could not convince the head of the blood bank of this urgent necessity, suggested it might be better if I ran the Blood Bank myself. He quickly agreed.

Experts in blood and blood products, infectious disease specialists, immunologists and specially-trained nurses were all needed to combat the myriad of complications that could arise from chemotherapy treatment. This team approach spawned the concept of the oncology nurse, and since these procedures were carried out in ambulatory facilities, it gave rise to the present highly-specialized chemotherapy units. Few hospitals were equipped to deliver this type of specialized treatment, and word quickly spread that the Brigham was one of the few hospitals set up to do so.

The significant numbers of leukemia cases we accumu-

lated enabled us to carry out studies utilizing various combinations of drugs and treatment schedules. Many of the
referred patients were young adults. As a physician, I
learned to keep a certain emotional distance, but one couple
really touched my heart. I first saw this lovely young
woman a few months after she had graduated from college.
She was terribly ill, with a full-blown case of leukemia. She
was engaged to be married to a classmate and it was my
sad task to call her fiancé in and tell the young couple the
terrible news that she had acute leukemia. They were very
much in love and sick as she was, they decided to get
married and go on their honeymoon as planned. I did not
attempt to dissuade them but only pointed out the inevitable outcome. We treated her aggressively and she achieved
a partial remission. They had a lovely honeymoon and she
died shortly thereafter. Several weeks after her death, the
young husband came in to see me. He told me how grateful
they were for the few wonderful days they'd had together.
We ended the conversation weeping in each other's arms.

Some Diseases We Could Cure

Some of the nonmalignant diseases we encountered gave
us considerable difficulties. In the late 1960s and early
1970s, cases of aplastic anemia began to appear following
the administration of the antibiotic, chloramphenicol. This
antibiotic had been widely used for several years before
cases of aplastic anemia began to appear. Bill Dameshek
brought suit against both the doctors who administered the
drug and the manufacturer of the drug. When Bill died
suddenly in 1969, I inherited the cases. Fortunately the use

of chloramphenicol was quickly discontinued and I was no longer put in the awkward position of testifying against other physicians.

The diagnostic enigma of the enlarged spleen was another disease that gave us trouble. In these cases, there were often no clues in the peripheral blood and sometimes the bone marrow contained few cells. At that time, we lacked good non-invasive methods of identifying intra-abdominal and retroperitoneal lymph nodes, so exploratory laparotomy and splenectomy were often carried out to establish the diagnosis. Fortunately, we had an excellent surgeon in Dick Wilson and an outstanding Anesthesiology Department. We were always very careful about selecting candidates for splenectomy; as a result, over the years, I can only recall one case of a postoperative fatality due to intractable bleeding.

In many cases in which the spleen was greatly enlarged, the patient's bone marrow had been replaced by scarring or fibrosis. In that case, the function of the bone marrow would be taken over by the spleen, liver, and abdominal lymph nodes. While splenectomy did not cure these patients, it provided at least temporary relief from severe pain due to splenic infarct or helped decrease the intensive discomfort of a huge bulky spleen. Unfortunately, the underlying disease persisted and eventually resulted in the death of the patient.

A Good Friend

Our referral practice grew faster than our space could accommodate, even taking into account successful forays into Dr. Wilson's exam room. Chemotherapy patients would crowd the waiting room and the exam room and overflow into the hallways. I.V. bags were set on tops of file cabinets, or attached to hangers suspended from the ceiling. Into this scene one day appeared Mac Hecht, an impressive middle-aged man. He was a trustee of the Children's Hospital and had been sent to us for treatment of CML.

We treated him with Busulfan, which required regular visits for blood counts and checkups. About his third visit, the waiting room was crowded and we were administering some medication to a patient with the I.V. apparatus hanging off one of the filing cabinets. After I finished with Mac, he made the astute observation that we really should have more room and better facilities. I agreed with him heartily, and he suggested I go see Gene Braunwald and request more space. Dr. Braunwald had recently taken over as Chief of Medicine from George Thorn. When I visited Gene and he told me that the Renal Unit under John Merrill was moving to new quarters, freeing up a large area off the Main Pike. Mac and I inspected the area. It had several large rooms, offices, and a good waiting room. It would need some alterations and laboratory facilities, but I was delighted with it until Dr. Braunwald told me it would take $200,000 to fix the place up. Well, I figured that was the end of that. When Mac came by to see me, I told him the price. He took a deep breath, then said, "Well, I'll sell off a few more bonds!"

Mac didn't live to see us move into our new space. Instead of responding well with a good remission, he relapsed and developed a blast cell crisis within a few

months of his diagnosis. When he died, we lost a great
man and a true friend. Mac left a bequest to our Hematology Division and his wife, Amalie, helped my successor
Frank Bunn administer it. Amalie wrote, with her husband
Edward Kass, an outstanding biography of Thomas Hodgkin, the man who first described Hodgkin's disease. She
remained a great friend and supporter of our Division.

In 1968, David Rosenthal left to go into the service for
two years. Fortunately, Arthur Skarin, who had been a
medical resident with me at BCH, was discharged from the
Air Force and at my urging joined me in Boston. Arthur
was a splendid doctor and had a distinguished career in
oncology/hematology. He and his wife, Roz, became our
close friends.

The Jimmy Fund

Though in theory I was Chief of Hematology at the Jimmy
Fund, and had a large office in the Jimmy Fund building to
back up the title, I didn't spend much time there; there were
simply too few adult cases of leukemia. Besides, Sidney
had a hoard of Fellows, mostly foreign, who were there to
do his bidding. Some of these people were good, others
pretty terrible, and I was openly critical of them.

The lab staff at the Jimmy Fund was not much better.
I had grown accustomed to the high level of competence
and professionalism we'd established at the PBBH. The lab
at the Jimmy Fund did have one excellent chief technician,
but the remaining technicians did not work well with her.
The result was a lackadaisical atmosphere, where work was
done slowly, if at all. One day I ordered a blood count for

a child. We couldn't administer any medicine until we got the lab results, so I ordered it "stat." We waited and waited. Finally I went myself to check on it, and found the technicians reading newspapers. I exploded and really chewed them out.

One of these technicians was a friend of Dr. Farber's secretary, whom we secretly called the "dragon lady." She of course relayed the information to Dr. Farber, and the next thing I knew I was on the carpet explaining to him that I did not take that kind of nonsense from technicians. I won the battle but could see I was losing the war. This was the beginning of what would be an ongoing feud between us.

Sidney Farber was a fine man, an outstanding leader in the field of oncology, and an excellent pathologist, but he had no clinical training. Yet he made all the decisions, and did not like to be challenged. My outspokenness did not sit well with Dr. Farber. Our relations continued to deteriorate until one day, in a conference of about forty people, Dr. Farber ordered me out. I was enraged, embarrassed, humiliated, and vowed I would never go back.

It was Jo who insisted I go back, reminding me how instrumental Dr. Farber had been in my career, and how he'd helped me get the large institutional grants, as well as the appointment to the Brigham Hospital. I took her advice and the next day went to see him. While I didn't apologize, I did explain my point of view. We settled our issues as amicably as we could, and agreed that, since I already had my job at the PBBH, I would leave the Jimmy Fund. I walked out of his office satisfied I'd done all I could. Dr. Farber died a week later, while seated at his desk.

Chapter Eleven

FROM HEYDAY
TO MAYDAY

1974–1997

W HEN THE Hematology Division moved to the third floor of the A building, Bob Handin's new office was three times the size of Frank Bunn's. I knew this indicator, though subtle, marked the beginning of the end for hematology as I knew it.

In 1974 I was made Professor of Medicine at Harvard Medical School. One year later I reached the age of sixty-six and had to retire, yet contined to stay involved. Three days a week I drove up from Chatham to review bone marrow slides with fellows. I continued to do this, though on an increasingly reduced basis, until 1997.

New Blood

Dr. George Thorn retired in 1972 after thirty years, and Eugene Braunwald was brought in as his replacement. David Rosenthal stayed on as Chief of Clinical Hematology and H.F. (Frank) Bunn, who succeeded me as Division Chief, created a whole new atmosphere of clinical research. Frank was a fine physician and a distinguished scientist. He had been a protege of Bill Castle and Jim Jandl at the Thorndike, and subsequentally became a productive clinical investigator, making major contributions in hemoglobin and red cell biology. When Frank came to see me prior to accepting the position at the Brigham, he was very humble. He came into my office, sat down and said he wanted to learn from me how to take care of patients with hematologic malignancies. I was somewhat overwhelmed by his kindness. As we worked together over the years we became close, and I now count Frank and his wife Betsy among my dearest friends.

With Dr. Braunwald's encouragement, Frank Bunn established research laboratories and tackled fundamental problems on a molecular level. At the same time, W. H. (Hal) Churchill, who had come to the Division as a fellow from the Massachusetts General, developed an interest in blood banking and became the Director of the Blood Bank. Joel Rappeport, formerly a resident in medicine at the Beth Israel Hospital and at the Boston City Hospital, joined the Division as a fellow and developed an interest in bone marrow transplantation. Working in this difficult field would have discouraged most individuals, but not Joel. He was one of the hardest working and most compassionate members of our Division, and he went on to create a bone marrow unit at Yale under Bernard Forget.

Not one of our senior people, including myself, David Rosenthal, Frank Bunn, or Bob Handin, was interested in solid tumors. The field of oncology was not very attractive to most physicians since there were few useful chemotherapeutic agents available; to this day there is still not a good chemotherapeutic solution. Surgery and radiation remain the only useful methods of treatment.

The Big Business of Cancer

With the arrival of Tom Frei and George Canellos at the Dana-Farber Cancer Institute, the adult cancer program rapidly expanded. The inpatient beds were all in the newly built Brigham and Women's Hospital, while greatly expanded ambulatory programs were conducted at Dana-Farber. Later, when David Rosenthal left to become Chief of the Harvard University Health Services, Bob Handin moved the Division to the field of solid tumors and Larry Shulman, trained in oncology, became the Clinical Director of the now combined Hematology-Oncology Division. This was a major shift for our division, and necessitated a large increase in outpatient facilities, along with an increase in in-patient admissions to the present Brigham and Women's Hospital. The staff had to be expanded, and emphasis began to shift away from studying the peripheral blood and bone marrow preparations.

The emphasis was on oncology because that was, and is, more profitable. Staff got so busy caring for the oncology patients that they no longer had time to come and look at bone marrows. I used to have a waiting list of people wanting to take the Bone Marrow Course; then I had no one. The priority, and the prestige, went to the molecular biologists.

Rats Die but Research Lives On

In spite of being officially *emeritus*, I still worked in much the same capacity, and continued diligently with my rat leukemia research. Unfortunately, the only prevalent form of leukemia in the rat was a strange disease which in some inbred strains of rats occurred spontaneiously in 30 to 40% of old rats. The cells appeared to be large mononuclear cells, and often the cytoplasm contained large blue granules. Actually, these were L.G.L. or large granular leukocytes, or "killer cells". They did not conform to the category of B or T cells; neither were they myeloid or monomyeloid in character. Since the leukemia did not have a human prototype, it proved useless experimentally.

However, by this time Joel Greenberger had become heavily involved in growing cells in culture and I collaborated with him in many of his experiments. We copied, from a Latvian investigator, a method of growing cells in diffusion chambers. These diffusion chambers were small collar button-like chambers made from silicone rings. Each side of the ring was sealed with a special filter which allowed free passage of liquids, but not cells, into the diffusion chamber. These chambers, four to six at a time, were introduced to the rat's peritoneal cavity. The rat had previously been heavily irradiated so that any immune response was eliminated. The chambers were removed on day one, three, seven and fourteen, and occasionally much later. The contents were removed, resuspended in serum, stained with Wright Giemsa stain, and then examined under the microscope.

In this way, cells from normal humans and patients with

various forms of leukemia or allied disease could be studied. In addition, the recipient rats could be treated with a variety of agents including erythropoietin and other growth-stimulating or growth-regulating factors. We carried out hundreds of experiments and found that normal bone marrow cells would grow from one to three days, then would be replaced by macrophages. Cells from untreated cases of AML proliferated actively in the diffusion chamber, after surviving without maturing for thirty or more days. Cells from patients with treated AML failed to survive more than one to three days. A great variety of other observations were carried out including histochemical and cytogenetic studies.

Research Dies Too

It was a great disappointment when, in 1982, Bob Handin called me into his office and told me I would have to give up this research program due to lack of funds. I believed the work we were doing was important. On the other hand, I recognized that, at my age, I could not expect to obtain research grants. Since I had not enticed younger fellows to work with me in this field of research, I agreed with Bob that my research should come to an end. Bob then said that he and Gene Braunwald wanted me to stop conducting rounds on the hematology patients, even though many of the patients had been referred to me personally. He said that the younger fellows felt that they should conduct the rounds and have more to say in diagnosis and treatment.

As a final straw, Bob went on to say that I should continue working as a consultant, but without salary. He thought it time I began to be supported by my pension and other retirement funds. This made me angry and I stood up and walked out of his office. My office was only a few doors down the hall and shortly thereafter came a knock on my door. Bob came in looking rather red-faced and worried. He'd obviously had a change of heart. He said he was sorry, then told me that he would not be in the position he was if it were not for my support and help.

We both calmed down, shook hands and parted amiably. The next day, Bob came up with an excellent suggestion. He wanted me to take over all the bone marrow readings, write a report for the record, and discuss the interesting cases with the housestaff, fellows, and associates. We averaged about 500 specimens a year and, in addition, read the special stains such as for iron, peroxidase, specific and nonspecific esterase, and the PAS stains. These histochemical stains were used to distinguish cytoplasmic enzymes, chiefly in leukemia cases, enabling us to more accurately classify the type of cell. Hitherto, the marrows were read haphazardly by residents or hematology fellows; the slides were not properly filed and the reports were poorly made out. So, I began in 1982 to read the bone marrows for the Division. The patient was charged $25.00 for each marrow specimen report, and I did upwards of 500 reports per year. In this way, I felt I more than carried my weight financially.

Hematology Bows to Oncology

I had a narrow, defined role within the hematology division. From this stable vantage point, I watched the changes in the division occur at a breakneck pace. There was a large contingent of fellows with hematology experience who were training to become oncologists. The new PhD/MD programs and availability of advanced training in molecular biology, genetics and other preclinical fields through the NIH fellowships improved the calibre of candidates. Salaries for interns, residents and fellows increased dramatically, enabling young medical students to continue their training in hematology/oncology.

David Rosenthal, now a Professor in the Harvard School of Public Health, only came one day a week to the Hematology Division. The new Chief of Clinical Hematology and Oncology, Larry Shulman, was primarily an oncologist and was interested mainly in solid tumors. The patient census rapidly rose along with a great increase in the ambulatory clinics for chemotherapy. Actually, the hematology/oncology fellows were too busy to participate in much else than admitting and taking care of patients on chemotherapy protocols. Frank Bunn stayed away as much as he could from the solid tumors; he and Hal Churchill, along with several older fellows, took care of the dwindling numbers of hematology patients. Their numbers declined as more and more cancer patients were enrolled in the program. Nonetheless, there were sufficient cases of blood diseases to provide for the training program's needs. However, it was a very obvious and disturbing fact that oncology was going to take over the hematology program.

In 1990, Bob Handin once again called me into his office and requested that I stop reading the bone marrows with the fellows. I was moved out of my office on the main floor into a large, odd-shaped room that extended out over the roof of the old "B" building. The office was at the end of a long corridor, up a small flight of stairs upon which were often stored boxes of books. There was a double set of steel doors to pass through, the first of which warned "This door should remain locked at all times." The interior door locked behind me, and I used to worry that one day I'd forget the key and be trapped up there for days. The office adjoined the building's main air-conditioner unit, a particularly noisy contraption that would have drowned out my pleas for help. Of course, I could always use my telephone to call for help, but more often than not the phone didn't work. I tried not to take it personally, and appreciated Bob Handin's generosity at continuing my part-time salary along with parking privileges and office privileges.

But Students Are Forever

Perhaps hearing I now had more free time than I'd like, Dr. Geraldine Pinkus, Chief of the Heme-Pathology Section, asked if I'd review the bone marrow specimens for her department. This was a great break for me. It allowed me to reduce my visits to twice per month while retaining some involvement in the program. Gerry attracted the best and the brightest of the pathology residents and fellows; the best part of working with this new group was that they had yet to hear my stories.

Students have always been an important part of my life, and the practice of hematology allowed me to work side by side with them throughout my career. It was the ideal specialty for me. Hematology provided the opportunity to teach, to contribute some important research, and to make a real difference in the lives of my patients. These are the ingredients that have made my career so meaningful. It was a blessed combination. It is the one recipe missing from *A Hematological Cookbook*. In my view, it is the most important one.

INDEX

Adams, Lane, 158
AIDS, 163
Alcoholism, 5–6
Alinginas atoll, 144
Allan, George, 28
American Cancer Society, 151, 153–
   154; Research supported by, 154–
   157; W. C. Moloney's work on
   behalf of, 152, 154, 157–158, 161,
   163
American Federation for Clinical
   Research, 38–39, 82–83, 166
American Medical Association, 9
American Society for Clinical Inves-
   tigation, 83, 131
American Society of Hematology,
   131
Amos, Harold, 156, 159
Anemia, 16–17, 29, 31, 69. See also
   Aplastic anemia; Hemolytic ane-
   mia; Pernicious anemia; Sickle
   cell anemia

Anesthesia, 23, 173
Antibiotics, 12, 28, 88. See also
   Chloramphenicol; Penicillin
Aplastic anemia, 119, 172
AraC, 170
Army Medical School, 35
Atomic bomb, 90; Medical effects
   of, 90–92
Atomic Bomb Casualty Commis-
   sion, Genetics Department, 101–
   103; Growth and Development
   Department, 101; Hematology
   Department, 101; Japanese resent-
   ment of, 103–104; And negative
   publicity in U. S., 103–104; Pa-
   thology Department, 101; Pediat-
   ric Department, 101; Statistics
   Department, 97; W. C. Moloney
   as Director of Hematology at,
   61, 89, 90–92, 96–100, 105–108,
   116
Atomic Energy Commission, 91, 109

Atomic radiation, 136, 144, 146–148, 150–151; And birth defects, 101–103; And Chernobyl accident, 111–112, 113, 150; And leukemia, 89, 97–100, 102, 105–107, 108, 111–113, 138, 139; In Marshall Islands, 143–148, 150–151; And neutron flux, 100–101; Relationship to cancer, 101–103; And Three Mile Island incident, 110–111. See also Radiation

Baltimore, David, 163
Beard, Joseph, 161
Beck, William, 123
Beth Israel Hospital, Boston, 63, 156, 178
Betty Lea Stone Fellowship Foundation, 156
Biguria, Fernando, 70, 87, 116
Bikini atoll, 110, 144, 150
Black-Schaffer, Bernard, 101
Blood, Cell proliferation, 122–123; Coagulation, see Coagulation; Donations during World War II, 37–38; Red cell cycling, 122–123; Storage of, 34; Typing, 57, 58
Blood, 99, 106, 131
Blood banks and banking, 34, 67, 68, 116, 171, 178
"Blood Club," 135
Blood plasma, 35–36, 48–49, 77, 78
Blood transfusion, 23, 25, 48–49, 57, 67
Blount, Sir Anthony, 151
Boice, John, 112
"Boloney virus," 128–129
Bond, V. P., 112, 145

Bone marrow, 29–30, 87, 119–120, 122, 167, 173, 179, 182, 184; Shift away from study of, 179; Transplantation of, 111–112, 124–125, 166; And W. C. Moloney's analysis of, 29–30, 119–120, 167, 182, 184; William Moloney Bone Marrow Course, 131–132, 167–168, 179
Boston, Irish in, 15, 16
Boston City Hospital, 1, 3, 17, 28, 29, 61, 65, 68, 70, 71–73, 74, 82, 85, 89, 169, 178; Mallory Institute of Pathology, 71, 86, 130; Mary E. Curley Building, 69; Sears Surgical Pavilion, 117; Tufts Hematology Laboratory, 117, 165–166; Tufts Medical Service at, 72–73, 74, 87, 165; W. C. Moloney as Chief of Laboratories at, 116–119, 130, 131, 164, 175
Boston College, 152
Boston Dispensary, 70
Boston Globe, 140
Boston Home for the Insane, 3
Boston Latin School, 2
Boston Medical Library, 83
Boston University Medical School, 21, 24, 72, 155, 156, 165; W. C. Moloney offered clinical professorship at, 69–70
Braunwald, Eugene, 174, 177, 178, 181
Brecker, George, 87, 135
Brigham and Women's Hospital, 116, 140, 179. See also Peter Bent Brigham Hospital
British Army Medical Corps, 108

British Medical Society, 84
Brookhaven National Laboratory, 111
Brown, Tom, 12, 27–28, 75
Bulletin of Atomic Scientists, 110
Bunn, Betsy, 71, 178
Bunn, H. Franklin, 73, 177, 178, 183
Burger, Dr., 105
Busulfan, 122, 174
Bywaters, Eric, 37–38

Cambridge City Hospital, 68, 73
Cambridge University, 151
Cancer, Effect of atomic radiation on, 111–113; Effect of radiation on, 112; Radioisotopes as therapy in, 117–119; Stigma attached to, 153; Tobacco link to, 153. See also American Cancer Society
Canellos, George, 170, 179
Carney, Andrew, 15
Carney Hospital, W. C. Moloney on staff of, 15–17, 25, 29, 31, 62, 63, 68, 82, 85
Castle, William B., 17, 67, 71, 178
Catholicism, W. C. Moloney's attitude toward, 3, 16, 62–63
Center for Disease Control, 140
Cerebrospinal meningitis, 43
Chain, Sir Ernst B., 43–44
Chemotherapy, 122–123, 133–135, 157, 170–171, 174, 178–179, 183; Combined program of, 133–135, 170–171
Chernobyl accident, 111–112, 113, 150
Children's Cancer Research Foundation, 156

Children's Hospital, Boston, 18, 78, 129, 167, 174
Chloramphenicol, 172, 173
Christian, Henry A., 37, 82
Christopher, Alice, 157
Christopher, Paul, 156, 157–159, 161
Churchill, W. H. (Hal), 178, 183
Cirrhosis, 77
Coagulation, 75, 76; Anti-coagulants, 80–81; Defect in, 26, 27, 78
Cocoanut Grove Night Club, Boston, 36
Cogan, David, 100
Cohn, Edwin, 177
College of Physicians and Surgeons of Boston, 21
Conlin, John, 165
Conrad, R. A., 145
Coombs, Robin, 1, 57, 59, 67, 83, 84; Coombs' test, 1, 59
Coumadin, 26
Crick, F. H. C., 161, 162
Cronkite, Eugene P., 36, 87, 111, 112, 145
Crosby, William, 134
Curley, James Michael, 22, 69
Cushing, Archbishop, 66

Dale, Sir Henry, 44
Dam, Henrick, 25, 27
Dameshek, William, 7, 31, 62, 84, 120, 131, 134–135, 172
Dana-Farber Cancer Research Foundation, 156, 170, 179
Daunarubacin, 170
Denny-Brown, Derek, 71
Desforges, Jane, 74, 76, 116
DeVita, Vincent, 133

Diamond, Louis, 68, 78
Dmochowski, Leon, 161
DNA, 171
Dunphy, J. Engelbert, 124–125
Durham, C. L., 145

Einewetock atoll, 150
Emory University Medical School,
  37
English, Martin J., 68–69
Erythropoietin, 122
Eyquem, A., 85

Factor V, 76, 77, 79
Farber, Sidney, 129–130, 165, 166,
  175, 176
Faulkner Hospital, 9, 17, 60, 164;
  W. C. Moloney on staff of, 24,
  62, 68, 166
Fibrinogen, 76, 78, 79
Fibrinogenopenia, 78–79
Finland, Maxwell, 71
Fleming, Sir Alexander, 44–45
Flexner, Abraham, 19–20, 21
Florey, Howard W., 43
Folic Acid, 126, 130, 132
Forget, Bernard, 178
Fort Bragg, 39, 40
Fort McPhearson, 38, 39
Frei, Emil, 135
Frei, Tom, 179
Fuchs, Klaus, 151
Fuller, Peter, 155, 156, 158

Gale, Robert Peter, 111–112
Galway Medical School, 84, 86
Gallo, Robert, 163
Garabedian, John, 115–116
Gardner, Frank, 80, 166

Gavin, James, 84
Georgetown Medical School, 73
Gofman, John, 141–142
Grady Hospital, 37
Greenburger, Joel, 169–170, 180
Gross, Eric, 161

Hachiya, Michihiko, 108–109
Haddow, Alexander, 122
Hall, Tom, 129, 134
Hamilton, Leonard, 138, 184
Hammer, Armand, 111
Handin, Robert, 177, 178, 179, 181–
  182
Harrington, William (Bill), 73, 74–
  75, 77, 80, 83, 86–87, 126
Harvard Medical School, 2, 15, 16,
  24, 35, 72, 155, 158–159, 177; De-
  partment of Pharmacology, 130;
  Department of Physical Chemis-
  try, 77
Harvard School of Public Health,
  183
Hellman, Samuel, 155–156, 169, 170
Hecht, Mac, 174–175
Hematology, Advances in 1930s, 24–
  30; Taken over by oncology, 182–
  183; W. C. Moloney's early
  interest in, 16–17; W. C.
  Moloney's early practice in, 29–30
Hematopoiesis, 87
Hemolytic anemia, 74, 119
Hemophilia, 77
Heparin, 81
Hiroshima, 89, 90–91, 92, 95, 97,
  98, 100, 103, 104, 105–106, 109
Hiroshima Medical School, 96–97
Hodgkin, Thomas, 175
Hodgkin's disease, 115–116, 119,

120–121, 138, 169, 175; Combined chemotherapy in, 133; Nitrogen mustard in treatment of, 121

Holland, James, 135

Holy Ghost Hospital, Boston, 73, 124, 126; W. C. Moloney as Chief of Medicine at, 64–67; W. C. Moloney's research at, 130

Home for Destitute Catholic Children, 3

Hungerford, L., 132

Huntington Memorial Hospital for Cancer Research, 159

Hydrogen bomb, 109–110, 136–137, 143–144, 151

Ideopathic thrombocytopenia purpura (ITP), 119

Ingelfinger, Franz, 165

International Agency for Research, Etiology of Cancer project, 112

International Society of Hematology, 76, 81, 83–84, 131

Iron deficiency disease, 16, 17

Isotopes, 117–119

Jacob, Stanley, 124, 125

James, Jerry, 86

Jandl, James, 178

Janeway, Charles, 78

Jaundice, 28; Hemorrhagic factor in, 27

Jimmy Fund, 129, 167, 175–176

Johns Hopkins Medical School, 23, 56

Johnson, Ralph, 140

Journal of Laboratory and Clinical Medicine, 75

Journal of the American Medical Association, 12

Journal of the Irish Medical Society, 85

Kark, Robert, 29

Kass, Amalie (Hecht), 175

Kass, Edward, 175

Kastenbaum, Marvin, 106

Kelleher, Frank, 108

Kelly, Patrick, 142

Kennedy, John, 84, 85, 86

Kenney, John, 117, 123

King, Vincent, 126

Kings County Hospital, Brooklyn, 4–7

Knowlton, Edward A., 20

Koagulation vitamin, 25

Koonz, Colonel, 38–39

Kracke, Roy, 37

Krumbhaar, E. B., 149

Kwajalein Island, 144, 145, 147, 148

Lancet, 139, 140

Landsteiner, Karl, 24, 25

Lange, Robert D., 99, 105–106

Lavin, James, 157

Law Review, 142

Lawson General Hospital, Atlanta, 36–38, 40

Leukemia, 31–32, 85–86, 87–89, 121–122, 137, 138; Adult form, 132–133; "Blast cell crisis," 122; Chemotherapy in, 134; Childhood form, 132–133; Childhood versus adult, 132–133; Effect of atomic radiation on, 89, 97–100, 102, 105–107, 108, 111–113, 138; Effect of ionizing radiation on,

Leukemia *(continued)*
112; Effect of radiation on 112,
113, 122, 137, 138; Progress on in
1950s and 1960s, 132–133;
SALES committee and, 161–163;
W. C. Moloney's interest in, 31–
32, 85–86, 87–89, 97–100, 105–
107, 108, 111–113, 114, 119,
128–129, 171–172; W. C.
Moloney's research on, 123–128,
180–181
Levine, Philip, 25, 83, 84
Life magazine, 103, 104
Long Island Medical School, 4–5
Lung cancer, 153
Lymphoma and lymphosarcoma,
119, 169
Lyons, Dr., 139

McCarthy, Joseph R., 151
Maclean, Donald, 151
Majuro Island, 147
Malaria, 74
Mallory Institute of Pathology, 71,
86, 130
Manchester Guardian, 110
Marshall Islands, 110, 113, 143–148,
150–151
Massachusetts, Division of Health,
64; Registration of physicians in,
19–22
Massachusetts Eye and Ear Infir-
mary, Boston, 100
Massachusetts General Hospital, 24,
65, 83, 178
Massachusetts Institute of Technol-
ogy, 137–138, 155
Massachusetts Medical Society, 9, 20

Medicine, Quality of in 1930s, 17,
23–24; Reform in, 17–22
Melanoma, 10
Meningitis, 43
6-Mercaptopurine, 123
Merrill, John, 174
Merritt, H. Houston, 71
Meyer, Leo, 149
Middlesex Medical School, 21
Minot, George R., 17, 71, 122
Mitchell, Al, 41
Mobile Army Surgical Hospital
(MASH), 47
Moloney, Billy (son), 35, 92
Moloney, Elizabeth (daughter), 35
Moloney, John, 128–129, 161, 162
Moloney, Josephine O'Brien (wife),
7, 8, 11, 23, 33, 35, 39, 40, 49,
50, 55, 60, 80, 89, 92–93, 98,
157, 176
Moloney, Patsy (daughter), 35, 39,
92
Moloney, Tommy (son), 34, 35, 98
Moloney, William C., Attends Inter-
national Society of Hematology's
meeting, Cambridge, 1950, 83–
84; As Atomic Bomb Casualty
Commission's Director of Hematology, 61, 89, 90–92, 96–100,
105–108, 116; And bone marrow
analysis, 29–30, 119–120, 167,
182, 184; As Boston City Hospital's Chief of Laboratories, 116–
119, 130, 164, 165; On Carney
Hospital staff, 15–17, 25, 27, 31,
62, 63, 82; And Catholicism, 3,
16, 62–63; College and medical
school training, 3–4; D-Day casu-

alties treated by, 47–54; Developing practice in hematology, 29, 30; Discovery of the "Boloney virus," 127–128; Early life, 1–2; Expert on radiation effects, 137–142; On Faulkner Hospital staff, 24, 62; "Hematological Cookbook" of, 1, 185; As Holy Ghost Hospital's Chief of Staff, 64–67, 86; Initial years in medical practice, 7–15; Interest in bleeding disorders, 77; Interest in hematology, 16–17; Interest in leukemia, 31–32, 85–86, 87–89, 97–100, 105–107, 108, 111–113, 114, 119, 128–129; 171–172, 180–181; Interest in medicine, 3–4; Interest in Rh factor, 25, 58, 59, 67–68, 70, 83, 84; Internship training, 4–7; Lack of surgical skill, 6–7; Leukemia research, 123–128, 180–181; Offered clinical professorship at Boston University, 69–70; Office in Back Bay, 30; Oversees radioisotopes at Boston City Hospital, 117–119; Participates in radiation fallout study in Marshall Islands, 145–148, 150–151; Participates on SALES committee, 161–163; As Peter Bent Brigham Hospital's Chief of Hematology, 166–176; Professor at Harvard Medical School, 177; Rejected as Chief of Medicine at St. Elizabeth's Hospital, 62–64; Retirement and retirement activities, 179–184; Stateside military service in World War II, 35–37; Teaches bone marrow course, 131–132, 167–168, 179; Trans-Atlantic crossing to England in World War II, 40; Trip to Japan, 1952, 93–94; Trip back from Japan, 1954, 109, 113–114; On Tufts Medical School faculty, 62, 70, 116, 130, 131; Wartime service in England before D-Day, 41–47; Witnesses hydrogen bomb explosion, 136–137, 142; Works on behalf of American Cancer Society, 152, 154, 157–158

Mononucleosis, 88, 119
Morgan, Ralph Z., 141
Murphy, William P., 17, 71
Mustogen, 133
Myeloma, 73, 83, 119, 139, 169
Myleran, 122

Nagasaki, 89, 91, 97, 98, 100, 103, 104, 106
National Cancer Institute, 133, 162
National Cancer Review, 112
National Institute of Health, 155, 169
Nature, 86
Neas, Maynard, 147
Neel, James, 101–102
New England Journal of Medicine, 32, 74, 139, 164
New England Medical Center, 24, 70–71, 87, 89, 166; Boston Dispensary, 70; Pratt Diagnostic Clinic, 70, 71
New York Hospital, 6
New York Times, 161

Newborn, Hemorrhagic disease of, 28–29
Nightingale, Florence, 165
Nitrogen mustard, 121, 125, 133
Norwell, P. C., 132
Norwood Hospital, 29

Oak Ridge Institute for Nuclear Studies (ORINS), 117–118, 123
O'Hara, Dwight, 70
O'Hare, James, 35
Oncogenes, 163
Oncology, 67, 179, 184
Oncology nursing, 157, 158
Oncovin, 133
Owren, Paul, 76, 77, 79–80, 83, 84, 85

Pacelli, Cardinal Eugenio, See Pius XII
Panope Island, 147
Papanicolaou smear, 153
Paritol, 80–82
Pasteur Institute, 85
Patton, General George, 54, 55
Pearl Harbor, Bombing of, 34
Penicillin, 43–45
Pernicious anemia, 16–17
Peter Bent Brigham Hospital, 15, 24, 65, 164; Hematology Division, 166–169, 174–175, 177–178, 182; Hematology-Oncology Division, 179, 182–183; W. C. Moloney as Chief of Hematology at, 166–176
Philby, Kim, 151
Pick's disease, 13
Pinkus, Geraldine, 184

Pius XX, Pope (Eugenio Pacelli), 14, 85
Pneumonia, 12, 43
Poliomyelitis, 18, 92, 147–148
Pratt Diagnostic Hospital, 70, 71
Portsmouth Naval Shipyard, 139–140
Prednisone, 132, 133
Primaquine, 74
Procarbazine, 133
Proger, Samuel, 70, 87
Prothrombin, 26, 27, 75, 76
Purine, 123

Quick, Armand, 27; Quick test, 27, 28, 30, 75

Race, R. R., 57–58, 67, 83, 84
Radcliffe Infirmary, Oxford, 42
Radioisotopes, 117–119
Rafferty, Helen, 10–11, 61
Rathke, Herbert, 43
Radiation, And development of leukemia and cancer, 112–113, 122, 137, 138; Ionizing, 112, 137, 138, 139, 141; W. C. Moloney as expert on effects of, 114, 137–142. See also Atomic radiation
Radiation therapy, 121, 122, 155–156, 157, 169, 170
Rappaport, Joel, 178
Retinoic acid, 133
Rh factor, 24–26, 58, 59, 67–69, 70, 83–84, 86
Rickover, Hyman, 139
Rongelap atoll, 144–146, 148, 150
Rongerick atoll, 144
Roosevelt, Eleanor, 103–104

Rose Lathrop Home for the Cancerous Poor, 3
Rosenthal, David, 167, 170, 171, 175, 177–178, 179, 183
Rundles, Wayne, 135
Rysner, Hughes, 156

St. Elizabeth's Hospital, 71, 73, 78; W. C. Moloney rejected as Chief of Medicine at, 62–64, 69
St. Margaret's Hospital, 4, 13, 25, 67, 68
St. Mary's Infant Asylum, 3, 4
St. Paul, Michel, 85, 86
SALES (Special Animal Leukemia Etiology Studies) Committee, 161–163
Salk vaccine, 148
Sanger, Ruth, 57, 83, 84
Schull, William J. (Jack), 101–102
Science magazine, 103–104
Segal, Maurice, 165
Shay, Harry, 127
Shea, Stephen, 86
Shen, Shu Chu, 67, 126–127
Sherlock, Sheila, 86
Shmiskis, Stanley, 159, 160–161
Shulman, Lawrence, 179, 183
Sickle cell anemia, 74
Sisters of Charity, 64, 66
Skarin, Arthur, 175
Sloan-Kettering Memorial Hospital, 138
Smoking, 153
Social service, 157
Souter, Alexander (Sandy), 29
Spellman, Cardinal Francis, 59, 62, 85

Spellman, John, 59, 60, 62, 63, 64, 66, 85
Spellman, John, Jr., 59, 60
Spencer, Everett, A Society of Physicians, 20
Spleen, 125, 126
Spleenomegalia, 122, 173
Sprong, David, 56
Squibb Pharmaceutical, 80–82
Stead, Eugene, 37, 38
Stohlman, Frederick, 71, 74, 77, 81, 87, 122
Stokes Adams Syndrome, 11
Stone, Betty Lea (Mrs. Robert), 159, 161
Stone, Robert, 159
Stone Junior Research Fellowship, 159–160
Subbarow, Yellapragada, 130

Taylor, F. H. Laskey, 76, 116
Taylor, George, 56, 57–59
Taylor, Grant, 37, 38, 89, 90, 98, 99, 104, 105
Temin, Howard M., 163
Thomas, Lewis, The Youngest Science, 17
Thorn, George W., 168–169, 174, 177
Thorndike Memorial Laboratory, 29, 67, 68–69, 71, 75, 76, 80, 83, 118, 178
Three Mile Island incident, 110–111
Thrombin, 76, 78
Thromboplastin, 27–28
Time magazine, 14, 105
Tokyo, 94–95, 109
Truman, President Harry S., 91

Tufts College, 3
Tufts Medical School, 4, 21, 24, 63,
    65, 66, 69–70, 73, 74, 89, 130,
    131, 155, 166
Tyrosine kinase, 132

Union Carbide Company, 138
U.S. Armed Forces Medical Com-
    mittee, 136
U.S. Department of Energy, 137,
    139
U.S. Justice Department, 140
U.S. Naval Radiological Defense
    Laboratory, 144
U.S. Naval Research Institute, 144
University of Chicago, 128
University of Massachusetts Medi-
    cal School, 156, 170
University of Pittsburgh, 170
Utirik atoll, 144, 148, 149–150

Valentine, William N., 123
Vincristine, 133
Vitamin B12, 126
Vitamin K, 25–26, 27, 28–29, 30

Wald, Neil, 113
Walsh, Rev. Michael, 152
Walter Reed Hospital, Washington,
    D.C., 35, 49
Warren, Shields, 110
Watson, J. D., 161, 162
Weinberg, Robert, 163
Weiner, Alexander, 24, 25, 27, 58,
    83, 84
Weiss, Soma, 37, 71
Welch, Norman, 31, 63
Wellesley College, 74
Williams, Robert H., 71
Wilson, Richard, 164, 173, 174
Wiltshire, Eve, 123
Wintrobe, Maxwell, 26, 74, 76; He-
    matology—The Blossoming of a
    Science, 84
Wistar Institute, Philadelphia, 127
Woodbury, Lowell, 97

X-ray, As cause of leukemia and
    cancer, 112

Yale Medical School, 86, 178